John H. Bennett

The restorative treatment of pneumonia

John H. Bennett

The restorative treatment of pneumonia

ISBN/EAN: 9783742826954

Manufactured in Europe, USA, Canada, Australia, Japa

Cover: Foto ©Lupo / pixelio.de

Manufactured and distributed by brebook publishing software
(www.brebook.com)

John H. Bennett

The restorative treatment of pneumonia

THE

RESTORATIVE TREATMENT

OF

PNEUMONIA

I have issued this memoir with a view of bringing more prominently and more generally under the notice of my medical brethren the great practical importance of the questions concerned in the successful treatment of pneumonia by restoratives. It consists essentially of a table which appeared in the fourth edition of my "Principles and Practice of Medicine," published last April; of an extension of the statistical facts, and conclusions therein referred to; and a reply to the observations which several distinguished physicians have made on various points involved in the inquiry. I am induced to hope that its perusal will persuade hospital physicians and others to assist me in collecting carefully-taken cases of acute pneumonia, tabulated in the same manner as my own, whereby the advantages of the practice may be either confirmed or negatived by general experience. In this manner, it appears to me, might definitely be settled a long disputed and fundamental question in practical medicine.

J. HUGHES BENNETT.

EDINBURGH, *February* 1856.

CONTENTS.

✦

RESTORATIVE TREATMENT OF PNEUMONIA.

⁕ ⟶

It must be admitted by every intelligent mind that the only proof of any successful medical practice must be the actual cures that are effected by it. But simple as this proposition may appear to the uninitiated, it is well known in medicine that nothing is more difficult than to establish the real curative power of any particular plan of treatment. If a disease can be proved to get well of itself—that is, if in the vast majority of cases it go through a certain progress and terminate favourably—one of two things may happen—1st, A considerable number of remedies, however opposite in their mode of action, may each be extolled as the means whereby the result is occasioned, although they may all be inert; the recovery, in truth, being entirely owing to the powers of nature: 2d, No remedies whatever may be given—the disease may be left to itself—when the question will arise, under what management or conditions does it disappear in the shortest time? Several diseases may now be considered as generally getting well of themselves, among which, uncomplicated delirium tremens, hooping-cough, and erysipelas, may be cited as examples.

There are other diseases, however, which have hitherto been considered very dangerous to life, and in which a number of fatal cases have always occurred, under whatever system of treatment they have been placed. Among these is pneumonia, which, from its frequency, from the violent symptoms it occasions, and from the anxiety it invariably creates, must always command the attention alike of the public and of the medical practitioner.

With regard to this disease, long and careful observation, great accuracy in recording facts, and sufficient opportunity of observation, such as only a public hospital can furnish, are requisite to the satisfactory establishment of success in its treatment. Pneumonia has this advantage, however—viz. that its detection by the conjoined observation of functional symptoms and physical signs, is now rendered so certain, among skilled physicians, that the fallacies inherent in the diagnosis of many other affections are removed from it. On this account it has recently been made the subject of numerous observations in the public hospitals of this and other countries, and careful records have been drawn up of its progress and mortality, under different systems of treatment, so that discussion regarding it may be expected to yield more positive conclusions than those on any other disputed question in medicine. Under these circumstances, the results of my practice for the last sixteen years in the Royal Infirmary of Edinburgh appear to me worthy the attention of the profession ; inasmuch as, while most satisfactory as to recovery, they are based upon a series of recorded facts, the accuracy of which will, I think, not be disputed.

The following Table includes all the cases of acute pneumonia which have been admitted into the Clinical Wards of the Royal Infirmary under my care from the 1st of October 1848 to the 31st of January 1865. During this period my term of service was at first four months in the year, and then, on alternate years, six months and three months. I find that, altogether, I have treated cases in the wards for 75 months, or a computed period of 6¼ years. The Table presents the leading facts presented by the cases, so as to enable the reader to judge of the effects of the treatment employed. The columns indicate—1st, The number of the case ; 2d, The name of the patient—D marks a double case, and Uns. an unsatisfactory one as to the duration of the disease ; 3d, The age ; 4th, The previous health, whether good, bad, or in any way particularly affected ; 5th, The day of admission, counting from the rigor, which indicates the commencement of the disease ; 6th, The duration of the disease, or the commencement of the convalescent state, counting in days from the period when the rigor occurred ; 7th, The number of days in the hospital after admission, or, should the disease have commenced in the hospital, counting from the rigor ; 8th, The frequency and character of the pulse on admission ; 9th, The number and character of the respirations on admission ; 10th, The side of the chest, and extent of pulmonary tissue involved ; 11th, If complicated with other diseases it is marked by a X; 12th, The treatment; 13th, General remarks ; and 14th, The volume and page where the case may still be found. It must be remembered that the cases were not recorded in reference to any statistical inquiry, but are those drawn up by my clerks in the Clinical Wards, at the bed-side, in obedience to long-established usage. They vary greatly, therefore, in value, and in a few the information on certain points required is defective. This is indicated in the Table by a note of interrogation.

The Table was commenced by my former able resident physician, Dr. Glen, whose early death, as medical superintendent in the Dundee Infirmary, in 1863, deprived the profession of a singularly well-informed and highly-educated physician. It was continued by Drs. Smart, Duckworth, and Macdonald, also my resident physicians in the Infirmary during the years 1863, 1864, and 1865, to whom I am greatly indebted for the pains they bestowed upon it. The fact that the Table has been constructed and carefully revised, not only by myself, but by each of these four gentlemen in succession, affords the most convincing proof of the accuracy of its details.

TABULAR VIEW of all the Cases of ACUTE PNEUMONIA treated in the Clinical Wards of the Royal Infirmary by the Author, from 1st October 1848 to 31st January 1865, while on service for 75 months, or a compiled period of 6¼ years.—Average number of Beds, 40.

MALE CASES.

No.	Name	Age	Previous Health	First seen after rigor. Days	Convalescence after rigor. Days	To Hospital. Days	Fever. At commencement of Treat. Total	Inspiration at commencement of Treatment.	Extent, and side involved.	Complicated.	Treatment.	Observations.—As to Nature of the Disease—Kind of Complication—Violence of Symptoms—Peculiarity of Physical Signs—Sequela, etc. etc.	Reference to Record in Hospital Case Books. Ward I.
1	J. Alhannan	30	Winter cough for 3 years	8	10	33	211	20, laboured	¾ lower R.S.		Bled before admission—amount not stated. Antimonials (1-10 gr. every 2d hour) Bitter afterwards. Wine ʒvj, and nutriment.	A strong labourer, with slight plenrity, and subject to cough in winter. After bleeding entered the house exhausted.	Vol. 3, p. 98.
2	R. King	40	Good	7	14	30	112, hard	Short	½ lower R.S.		Not to get after admission by Clerk. Antimonials (2-3 gr. every hour). Afterwards tonics. Bitters.	Entered a weak after attack. Was bled and antimonialised.	Vol. 3, p. 6
3	J. Foreman	34	Good	4	8	17	100, full and strong	Dyspnœa	⅔ lower L.S.		Antimony 1 gr. every hour. Afterwards expectorant mixture, nutriment and porter.	A strong man—entered soon after attack. Not exhausted.	Vol. 4, p. 141
4	J. Kell	40	Good	4	14	18	100, good strength	Hurried and alert	¾ lower L.S.		Antimony 1 gr. every two hours—then every hour. Afterwards opiates to procure sleep, and gill of whisky daily.	A strong plethoric man, addicted to drink.	Vol. 4, p. 106
5	J. M'Intyre	59	Good	14	21	30	96, good strength	Dyspnœa	1 lower L.S.		Antimony 1 gr. every hour—afterwards 1-10th gr. every fourth hour, combined with nutrients. Subsequently tonics.	Convalescence commenced soon after admission, but was prolonged	Vol. 5, p. 116
6	D. Hogg, D 1	18	Weak	14	35	54	Natural	No dyspnœa	Both S. 1		Bled, purged, blistered, sq., before admission. Saline, wine ʒiv, nutrients, Arthingtons and opiates afterwards to check diarrhœa.	A weak young man, a teacher, treated antiphlogistically before admission, and convalescence further lengthened by supervening diarrhœa.	Vol. 6, p. 93
7	S. Purcell	58	Good	4	22	36	100, full and hard	Dyspnœa	⅔ upper R.S.		⅓ gr. antimony every third hour; wine ʒiv; nutrients.	Disease is first-noticed in middle third of right lung, and subsequently extended to upper third	Vol. 6, p. 128
8	W. Hamilton	33	?	2	14	32	100, full	Easy	¾ upper L.S.		Cupped to ʒviij. Antimony ½ gr. every four hours; wine ʒvj. Blister. Quinine 1 gr. thrice daily.	An uncommon diminished, prolonged expiration and sibilant rale appeared at apex, convalescence lengthened.	Vol. 7, p. 111
9	J. Conolly	30	Vigorous	6	14	34	90, full	?	1 lower R.S.		½ gr. anti. bext every three hours. Nutrients. Rheumatic pains treated by aconite locally.	On the recovery of this case there supervened an attack of rheumatism, which prolonged his stay in the house.	Vol. 3, p. 174

13

No.	Name		Constitution		Age	Duration	Pulse	Respiration	Side affected	Treatment	Remarks	Reference
10	R. Leich, D 3	13	Vigorous	4	14	14	194, strong	Easy	½ lower L, 3, ½ lower R, 3	Sallnes; blister; nutrimeta.	A strong young labourer, with strong pulse and rapid recovery, though both lungs were affected.	Vol. 8, p. 41.
11	J. Kelty	60	Not good.	14	20	21	73, natural	Oppressed	½ lower R, 3	Sallnes; vin. codebel; nutrimein.	A strong muscular-looking man, long subject to cough and rheumatism.	Vol. 8, p. 78.
12	J. Stewart	18	Vigorous	3	7	7	104, full and strong	Hurried	Whole of L. R.	Bled to ℥xij, to relieve dyspnœa. Afterwards 12 leeches applied. Sallnes; then nutrimeta and wine.	The bleeding relieved dyspnœa, but caused prolonged convalescence; the length of which is not stated.	Vol. 9, p. 194.
13	T. Monro	24	Weak and gouty	4	21	32	78, natural	?	½ lower R, 3	Pulv. opii gr. ss. every two hours. Nutrimein, wine.	A debilitated man of gouty habit, treated with opium.	Vol. 11, p. 39.
14	H. M'Phillips, D 3	10	Good	4	13	34	100, strong	34, difficult	½ lower L, 3, and ½ lower R, 3.	Antimony ½ gr. every third hour, combined with 1-5 gr. of opium to relieve sleeplessness and severe general pain.	This case was well 16 days before dismissal, and the cause of his detention is not stated.	Vol. 14, p. 141.
15	D. Tayler	42	Winter cough for 23 years	3	16	24	100, full and strong	Dyspnœa	½ lower L, 3.	× Antimony and opium every third hour.	Complicated with bronchitis and emphysema.	Vol. 14, p. 145.
16	A. Miller	64	Good	2	7	7	100, small and soft	dyspnœa	½ lower L, 3	½ gr. of antimony and opium every second hour.	A healthy man. Rapid recovery.	Vol. 14, p. 155.
17	W. Grey	17	Good	4	16	21	104, good strength	38, difficult	½ lower R, 3.	½ gr., afterwards increased to 1 gr., of antimony every third hour.	This patient was convalescent 14 days after admission, and the cause of his detention is not explained.	Vol. 17, p. 35.
18	R. MacDonald	25	Good	2	16	18	105, full	44, hurried	½ upper R, 3.	1 gr. of antimony every two hours. Afterwards ℥ leeches and a blister.	Detained in the hospital 6 days after complete recovery.	Vol. 18, p. 177.
19	J. Donaldson	20	Good	6	16	38	128, good strength	Hurried	½ lower R, 3.	× Sallnes; wine frill; and nutrimein.	Had recovered from the treatment 10 days after admission. Detained 14 days longer with continued fever.	Vol. 18, p. 31.
20	J. Scott	28	Ill four years	1	43	60	?	?	½ lower R, 3.	× Antimony ½ gr. every fourth hour. Cupped to ℥vi. Afterwards blister applied.	This was the fourth attack of pneumonia in four years. The former were treated antiphlogistically. Very slow convalescence with bronchitis.	Vol. 20, p. 108.
21	J. Leggat	10	Good	4	12	12	108, full	30, short	½ upper R, 3.	½ gr. antimony every hour; afterwards every second hour.	Vigorous young man. Rapid recovery.	Vol. 20, p. 34.
22	M. Mahon, Um. L	32	Good	8	4	29	165, full and strong	34	Whole of L. R.	Antimony ½ gr. every three hours; afterwards nutrimein.	A healthy boy, the date of whose convalescence, owing to absence of daily reports, could not be determined.	Vol. 21, p. 32.
23	J. Murray	53	Long cough	7	25	21	115, good strength	Dyspnœa	½ lower R, 3.	Antimony ½ gr. every two hours. Blisters, diaretics, ½j wine, and nutrimein.	Recovery delayed by chronic bronchitis.	Vol. 21, p. 145.
24	J. M'Naughton, D 4	34	Bad	6	21	34	100, weak	ill, difficult	½ lower on both sides	½ gr. of antimony every two hours twice, ℥vj wine, and nutrimein.	A weak man of intemperate habits. Entered the house exhausted. Recovery delayed.	Vol. 22, p. 133.

No.	Name	Age	Previous Health	First seen (Days)	Convalescence after illness (Days)	In Hospital (Days)	Pulse at commencement of Treatment	Manifestations at commencement of Treatment	Extent and Side involved	Convulsive	TREATMENT.	OBSERVATIONS.—As to Nature of the Case—Kind of Complication—Violence of Symptoms—Peculiarity of Physical Signs—Sequelæ, &c., &c.	Reference to Record in Hospital Case Books, Ward 1.
21	J. Bayliard	29	Very healthy	3	17	28	54 soft	24	½ lower L. B.		Diet before admission to Inf.; and purgat. ½ gr. of antimony and 4.5 Sol. Mur. Morph. every second hour.	A vigorous young man in perfect health. The bleeding relieved dyspnœa, but protracted convalescence.	Vol. 23, p. 141.
22	P. Clarke	23	Rather impaired	7	14	8	104 strong	Dynp-nœa	½ upper R. B.		¼ gr. of antimony every two hours; afterwards antichrist.	General health enfeebled by previous illness. He still made a good recovery.	Vol. 23, p. 1.
27	F. Geary (D.)	24	Cough for six weeks	5	16	53	112, soft	50	½ lower L. B.; upper R. B.		½ gr. antimony every four hours; cibaries; wine gill, and medicine.	Antimony caused diarrhœa and was discontinued. Detained a week after complete recovery.	Vol. 23, p. 164.
26	J. Proudfoot (D.)	30	Cough for six weeks	4	21	49	120, full and strong	22, diffi-cult	½ lower both sides		½ gr. of antimony every four hours. Wine and gin 34 gill, and medicine.	A man long addicted to whisky-drinking, with impaired health. Convalescence tedious.	Vol. 24, p. 137.
29	C. Enage	41	Rheumatic	2	15	37	86, good strength	1	Whole of R. B.		½ gr. of antimony every third hour. Enfeeblematic and afterwards astringents to check diarrhœa.	An intemperate man, with chronic rheumatism. Detained in the house with persistent diarrhœa.	Vol. 24, p. 6.
39	R. Simpson	33	Good	3	15	15	?	Tranquil	½ lower R. B.		½ gr. of antimony every three hours; afterwards stimulants and expectorants.	A simple case, in a healthy man, terminating in recovery on the 18th day.	Vol. 24, p. 108.
31	A. M'Naughton	27	Good	4	14	11	64, strong?	½ lower L. B.		½ gr. of antimony, and gill Sol. Mur. Morph. every four hours; whisky.	Natural progress of a simple pneumonia in a healthy man.	Vol. 25, p. 17.
32	J. M'Quair	19	Impaired	4	14	22	208, full	12, har-ried	Whole of R. B.		Diet twice before admission to Inf.; cibaries; antimony ½ gr., and subsequently ½ gr.; every third hour.	A disorganised youth with incipient phthisis. Convalescence retarded.	Vol. 24, p. 178.
33	B. Jade (D.)	55	Good	9	14	22	60, weak	39	½ lower both sides		Purgate enlarged before admission; antimony afterwards.	Recovery of appetite slow, and convalescence retarded.	Vol. 22, p. 148.
34	J. Cogsan (D.)	23	Good	4	18	30	96, strong	?	½ middle L. B., lower R. B.		Saline; wine gill, and nutrients.	Complicated with typhus fever, which prolonged convalescence.	Vol. 22, p. 161.
35	R. Macfarlane	20	Good	5	12	18	104, strong	24, easy	4-5th low-er L. B.		Saline; then diuretics with colchicum.	An ordinary case with good recovery.	Vol. 35, p. 3
36	A. Bathgate (D.)	22	Not good	7	18	34	120, full and hard	19	½ upper R. B., ½ upper L. B.	X	Saline; diuretics with colchicum; wine gin, and nutrients.	A debilitated intemperate man. The pneumonia on L. B. came on 7 days after that on R. B.	Vol. 25, p. 27.

No.	Name	Age	Habit								Site	Treatment	Result
38	P. Robertson D 10	51	Robust	4	11	9	100, weak		40		lower L. & lower L. S.	Nutrients and stimulants; wine $\bar{3}$iv; poulticed to L. S. Quinatic.	A strong man, with great dyspnœa and livid tinge of face threatening suffocation, which diminished in two days.
39	B. Beagle	38	Good	4	28	24	90, weak		Dry-gums	1 lower L. S.	Nut to $\bar{3}$xvij. Antiseptical treatment before admission. Intermittis wine $\bar{3}$ij, then $\bar{3}$v, Quinatic.	The treatment before admission led to prostration and prolonged convalescence.
40	J. Adams	40	Somewhat intemperate	4	14	12	110, small and weak		Much dyspnœa	2 lower L. S.	Beside; steak $\bar{3}$ij; and wine $\bar{3}$iij daily	In no estate at Glasgow 7 months before, was too ill, recertified, etc., and recovered slowly, with great weakness. On this occasion recovered rapidly.
41	G. Sanders	40	Intemperate	4	11	13	185, small and weak		80, tremulid	3 lower L. B.	Saline, nutrients, and wine $\bar{3}$ij.	A weak person.
42	Thornham	16	Good	8	14	4	100, soft		†	Whole of R. B.	Saline, wine $\bar{3}$iij, and nutrients.	This case now cannot be found—back missing.
43	T. Begley	40	Good	6	24	18	98, good strength		†	4 lower L. S.	Saline combined with stimulants; wine $\bar{3}$iv, and nutrients.	A simple case.
44	J. W Farhus D 11	39	Long subject to cough, asthma, and occasional haemoptysis	8	2	21	88, full and strong		40, dimcult	lower of L. S. and of R. S. apex.	At first, 1-18 gr. antim. tart. with zss and seps., and every six hours. Cupped to chest, and $\bar{3}$v of blood extracted to reduce dyspnœa. Afterwards $\bar{3}$v of wine daily with nutrients. Rheumatism treated by alkalies internally.	A tall, weak-looking man. Had rheumatic pains for ten years. All the symptoms became violent, and the physical signs well marked (on crepitatant cough, followed by crude consolidation, which prolonged his residence in the house.	X
45	Ed. Nugent	28	Good	2	?	?	90, weak		? internal	1 lower L. S.	Stimulants to reduce system and overcome collapse; then nutrients, and wine $\bar{3}$iv daily.	A strong healthy-looking man. Seized with sudden and great weakness. Entered the house one hour afterwards. Rallied by rest and stimulants. On the third day pneumonia established. Rapid and complete recovery.
Unit ?													
46	J. Tait	47	Drunkard	4	4	68	72, small and weak		1 great dyspnœa	4 lower L. S.	$\bar{3}$iv wine and $\bar{3}$ij of whisky in 24 hours. Nutrients as $\bar{3}$iij.	Detained in the house on account of chronic alcoholism and acute illness.
47	A. Robertson D 12	43	Weak & ill 16 months	14	10	36	112, weak		1 dyspnœa	4 upper both sides	Diuretics; $\bar{3}$iv wine, and nutrients.	Phthisical symptoms preceded attack, which disappeared.
48	J. O'Dennot	14	Good	6	22	13	130, weak		48	4 upper R. S.	Wine $\bar{3}$iv daily; liquid nutrients ad lib.; night saline.	The pneumonia was as at the apex, but resolved rapidly.
49	R. Kay D 13	35	Good	4	13	13	100, full and strong		40	lower L. & lower R. S.	Saline; nutrients; wine $\bar{3}$iv.	The pneumonia began and was most severe on the left side. There was a little pleurisy.

No.	Name.	Age.	Previous Health.	First Actual after Rigor.	Convalescence after Rigor.	In Hospital.	Pulse. At commencement of Treatment.	Respirations at commencement of Treatment.	Extent, and Side involved.	Complication.	Treatment.	Observations.—As to Nature of the Case—Kind of Complication—Violence of Symptoms—Peculiarity of Physical Signs—Sequelæ, etc. etc.	Reference to Record in Hospital Case Books. Ward 1.
				Days	Days	Days							
50	P. M'Elkim D 14	56	Good	5	10	20	90, good strength	28, oppressed	⅔ lower both sides		Salines; strong beef-tea; wine ℥iv, afterwards increased to ℥viij.	Dismissal delayed, from want of shoes and clothes, 12 days.	Vol. 45, p. 153
51	W. Purdie D 15	17	Good	2	16	13	120, full and soft	46, hurried	⅔ lower R. S., ½ lower L. S.		Salines; strong beef-tea; wine ℥iv.	Dismissal delayed for 2 days from want of clothes.	Vol. 46, p. 1.
63	W. Sword D 16	31	Good	7	15	16	96, weak	44	½ upper and lower M. S., ½ lower L. S.		Slight diuretics. Wine, at first, ʒi every two hours, with a teaspoonful of brandy to counteract perspiration; afterwards reduced to ℥iv daily. Strong beef-tea ad lib.	Very weak on admission; saved by stimulants.	Vol. 46, p. 23.
53	C. Hazard	34	Good	0	11	9	88, strong	48, laboured	Whole of R. S.		Salines; wine ℥iv; nutrients.	Strong vigorous man.	Vol. 47, p. 54.
64	J. M'Donald D 17	37	Good	3	8	11	108, fair strength	58, oppressed	⅔ lower L. S., ½ lower R. S.		Salines; wine ℥xij, afterwards diminished to ℥viij, with a little brandy.	Slight pleurisy of left side. Great exhaustion on 5th day, from which he was rallied by stimulants.	Vol. 46, p. 30.
55	J. M'Lauchlin	25	Good	4	8	10	88, fair strength	56, short	Whole of R. S.		Salines; nutrients; wine ℥ij.	Vigorous young man.	Vol. 47, p. 109.
66	J. Baker D 18	57	Bad	6	14	16	104, fair strength	56, urgent dyspnœa	Whole of R. S., ½ lower L. S.	X	Salines; diuretics; wine ℥viij.	Long subject to cough, palpitation, and dyspnœa. Rheumatism 9 years ago. Mitral regurgitation.	Vol. 46, p. 36.
57	F. Joyce D 19	19	Good	4	8	10	104, full and strong	48	⅔ lower R. S., ½ lower L. S.		Salines; nutrients; wine ℥iv.	Strong vigorous young man.	Vol. 46, p. 74.
58	F. Flinn	31	Good	5	8	7	104, weak	44, difficult	Whole of R. S.		Salines; nutrients; wine ℥iv.	A strong man, with rapid recovery. The disease occupied an entire lung.	Vol. 47, p. 65.
59	J. Lain	23	Good	4	7	12	96, fair strength	34, tranquil	⅓ middle R. S.		Salines; nutrients; wine ℥iv.	A vigorous young man, rapid recovery.	Vol. 45, p. 60.
60	J. Kitchen	47	Good	5	8	7	72, good strength	32, hurried	⅓ upper R. S.		Salines; diuretics; nutrients; wine ℥iv.	An intemperate man; delirium; good recovery.	Vol. 46, p. 38.
61	J. Durkin	40	Good	5	14	15	104, good strength	56, dyspnœa	⅔ lower L. S.		Salines; slight diuretics with colchicum; wine ℥vi; nutrients.	Very severe case.	Vol. 45, p. 157.

18	284, strong	dyspnœa	2 upper R. S.	Sallnce; strong beef-tea; wine &c.	No phthisis; made a complete recovery.	Vol. 44, p. 161.
30	64, full	38	3 lower L. S.	Sallnce; nutricals; wine &c.	Rapid recovery, ushered in with slight diarrhœa.	Vol. 43, p. 178.
73	58, feeble	—	3 upper L. S.	Sallnce; nutricals; wine &c.	No phthisis; made a complete recovery.	Vol. 43, p. 137.
30	102, weak	—	3 middle L. S., 3 L. S.	Sallnce; nutricin.	Bronchitis. Broncho-pneumonia.	Vol. 60, p. 77.
10	94, strong	—	2 R. S.	Sallnce, etc.; wine &c.	A strong vigorous man.	Vol. Lost.
81	108, good strength	Easy	3 lower L. S.	Sallnce; nutricals; wine &c.	Strong man. Typhoid fever will prolong slow convalescence.	Vol. 83, p. 31.
11	105, weak	48, dyspnœa	3 lower R. S.	Sallnce; nutricals; wine &c.	Simple case, recovering quickly. Slow convalescence.	Vol. 63, p. 73.
57	74, weak	30, dyspnœa	Whole of R. S.	Nutricals; wine &c.	Chronic pleurisy with effusion increasing daily; prior to admission. Complications except of pneumonia could not be determined.	Vol. 65, p. 68.
56	108, weak	30, dyspnœa	3 lower R. S., 3 upper R. S.	Sallnce; nutricals; wine &c.	A strong young man. Commenced on right side, will appear afterwards on left side.	Vol. 64, p. 98.
58	105, weak	42, urgent dyspnœa	Whole of R. S., 3 lower L. R.	Nutricals before admission to fair. Sallnce; nutricals; wine &c.	Extreme weakness. Slow convalescence. Dulness with slight compression of apex of right lung.	Vol. 64, p. 88.
44	118, weak	Short and Dulness	3 lower R. S.	Cupped and purged before admission. Nutricals; wine &c.	A case of typhoid fever, with abdominal. Slow recovery.	Vol. 65, p. 98.
55	68, weak	—	3 lower L. S.	Wine &c.; nutricals.	A man exhausted by a week's starvation before admission.	Vol. 65, p. 114.
32	104, weak	Dyspnœa	3 lower R. S.	Cupped before admission—to what extent unknown. Wine &c.; nutricals.	This is the same case as No. 71. Another attack. On admission still complains of apex of right lung.	Vol. 64, p. 233.
10	100, feeble	36, urgent dyspnœa	3 lower R. S., 3 lower L. S.	Nutricals; wine &c.	A vigorous young man. Rapid recovery.	Vol. 55, p. 109.
7	108, good strength	42, difficult	3 middle R. S.	Nutricals; wine &c.	Very slight pleurisy.	Vol. 65, p. 157.
52	84, weak	36	3 lower R. S.	Nutricals, etc.; wine &c.	Slight pleurisy with effusion.	Vol. 56, p. 7.
71	110, weak	34, dyspnœa	3 upper R. S.	Nutricals; wine &c.	Vigorous young labourer.	Vol. 57, p. 58.

No.	Name	Æ.	Previous Health.	First seen after Rigor. Days	Convalescence after Rigor. Days	In Hospital. Days	Pulse. At com-mencement of Sternal Pain.	Development at commencement of	Extent and Side involved.	Complicated.	Treatment.	Observation.—As to Nature of the Case—Kind of Complication—Violence of Symptoms—Peculiarity of Physical Signs—Sequelæ, etc. etc.	Reference to Record in Hospital Case Books. Ward 1.
79	Geo. Fleming	21	Not good	7	9	25	88, weak	30	½ lower L.B.	X	Nutrients; wine ʒiij.	The pneumonia followed a severe and prostrating attack of rubeola.	Vol. 57, p. 55.
80	John Devine	24	Good	7	10	8	89, weak	40, dyspnœa	⅓ lower R.B.		Nutrients; wine ʒvj.	A strong man—rapid recovery.	Vol. 57, p. 71.
81	A. Henderson	32	Good	6	13	12	86, full of good strength	34, no dyspnœa	½ lower L.B.		Moisture; wine ʒiv.	Strong healthy man. Diarrhœa on admission. Yeast-like stools up to ʒiij. with day from rigor.	Ward 10, vol. ..., p. ...
82	J. Walsh	42	Good	5	10	16	70, soft	37	½ lower L.B.		Salines; poultice to side; fʒj of wine for two days. Blister to side subsequently.	A healthy man, given to spirit-drinking. Formerly had pleuro-pneumonia.	Ward 1, vol. 59, p. 7K.
82	J. Duffin	19	Occasional bronchitis	6	9	10	100, strong	29	½ lower L.B.		Salines; beef-tea.	Much benefited, which completely disappeared.	Vol. 58, p. 78.
81	Mch. Drennan	10	Good	6	11	14	90, weak	34	⅓ lower R.S.		Salines; nutriments; ʒvj wine.	Much benefited. Enlarged by starvation previous to admission.	Vol. 58, p. 317.
83	John Dell	32	Good	5	12	16	98, fair strength	48, cyanpnœa	⅓ lower L.S.		Salines; nutriments; ʒviij wine.	Second attack of pneumonia. Health intemperate.	Vol. 60, p. 154.

FEMALE CASES.

No.	Name	Æ.	Previous Health.	First seen after Rigor. Days	Convalescence after Rigor. Days	In Hospital. Days	Pulse. At com-mencement.	Development at commencement of	Extent and Side involved.	Complicated.	Treatment.	Observation.	Reference. Ward 11.
84	S. Flynn Una. 5	14	Ill 3 months	0	7	18	138, small	Dyspnœa	⅓ lower L.B.		Diet to ʒiij on admission. 4 gr. antim. tart. every two hours.	Record defective. Commencement of convalescence cannot be determined.	Vol. 1, p. 78.
67	M. Dixon Una. 6	42	Ill 5 weeks	7	12	32	132, soft	†	⅓ lower R.B.		Salines; blister.	Commencement of pneumonia not stated.	Vol. 1, p. 131.
88	B. McCormack D 24	40	†	6	20	38	132, hard	Suppressed	⅓ lower R.S., ⅓ lower R.B.		¼ gr. antim. tart. every second hour; blister.	Previous health not stated.	Vol. 3, p. 60.
88	A. Connor D 75	9	Not good, debilitated	6	31	45	136, soft	Hurried	⅓ lower R.S., ⅓ upper R.S.		Tr. digital. mv every four hours; lemonade; afterwards ʒ lindin to side to relieve pain.	Great exhaustion and unusual action of the heart in this case.	Vol. 5, p. 265.
90	A. Donolly	39	Long had bronchitis	1	10	12	100, full	Dyspnœa	⅓ lower R.S.		8 leeches; 1 gr. antim. tart. every hour, with ½ gr. pulv. opii.	Strength good in this case on admission.	Vol. 5, p. 188.

91	M. Cowan Uns. 7	28	Cough and dyspnœa for 3 months	?	7	32	100, weak	Dyspnœa	½ lower R. S.		Wine ℥iv; ¼ gr. antim. tart. every four hours; 8 *leeches afterwards to relieve pain.*	The previous illness caused commencement of pneumonia to be undetermined.	Vol. 6, p. 183.
92	M. Carle	15	?	6	10	6	100, full	Dyspnœa	½ lower R. S.		12 *leeches to painful side;* ¼ gr. antim. tart. every three hours; blister.	Considerable pain in side—relieved by leeches.	Vol. 7, p.
93	M. Dickson	34	?	6	19	25	104, good strength	Urgent dyspnœa	½ lower R. S.		¼ gr. of antimony with ¼ gr. of opium to relieve pain; diuretics; subsequently 12 *leeches* and 2 blisters were applied.	Previous health not stated.	Vol. 8, p. 93.
94	R. White D 26	28	?	3	13	6	92, strong	Dyspnœa	½ lower Both sides		Salines; 8 *leeches* and blister; wine ℥vj.	Previous health not stated.	Vol. 9, p. 7.
95	S. Reynolds	26	?	5	16	28	120, full and strong	Hurried	½ lower R. S.		1 gr. antimony every two hours; discontinued after 24 hours; *afterwards* 12 *leeches were applied;* wine ℥vj; blister.	General health probably enfeebled by previous nursing. Very weak after subsidence of febrile symptoms.	Vol. 9, p. 110.
96	C. M'Donald	15	Cough for a month	1	10	35	120, soft and weak	36	Whole of L. S.		Salines; 6 leeches, and afterwards blisters were applied.	A simple pneumonia, with unretarded recovery. No indication for wine.	Vol. 11, p. 14.
97	M. Hodges	38	Good	7	16	23	60, strong and full	Difficult	Whole of L. S.		1 gr. antimony every four hours, and a blister applied to the side.	Rigors and cough, but no physical signs on admission. These appeared on 4th day.	Vol. 12, p. 40.
98	M. M'Donald	20	Feeble	10	18	24	66, weak	No dyspnœa	½ lower R. S.		Salines; ℥iij wine and nutrients, with ⅙ gr. of tartar emetic. Blister to right side.	Subject to occasional cough and pain in the chest before the attack.	Vol. 12, p. 119.
99	J. Smith Uns. 8	13	?	10	?	14	80, strong	?	½ lower R. S.		Salines and nutrients.	Had not been under treatment before admission, though ten days had elapsed since the rigor.	Vol. 13, p. 152.
100	H. Dalloch	16	Rheumatic	1	19	105	108, moderate strength	40	½ lower L. S.	X	¼ gr. of antimony every four hours; a blister; wine ℥iv, increased to ℥vj, and nutrients. Rheumatism treated with diuretics and anodynes.	Acute rheumatism and cardiac disease detained her in the hospital. Pleuro-pneumonia commenced two days after admission.	Vol. 14, p. 28.
101	M. Ross	30	Subject to coughs	3	16	58	104, weak	Laboured	½ lower L. S.		Salines with small doses of morphia; blisters; ℥viij wine.	Diarrhœa in the course of convalescence, which was prolonged.	Vol. 16, p. 74.
102	A. Smith	32	Weak	9	25	28	78, weak	?	½ lower L. S.		¼ gr. tartar emetic; 3 gr. calomel daily for a week; 4 *leeches;* salines; wine ℥vj; 7 *leeches;* nutrients.	In weak health previously. Period rather long before convalescence occurred.	Vol. 17, p. 128.
103	M. Corrigan	25	Good	4	14	10	96, strong	?	½ lower L. S.		Slight salines; blister applied; and wine ℥iij.	A simple pneumonia in a previously healthy woman.	Vol. 17, p. 168.
104	M. Kay	40	Not good	6	18	45	106, weak	?	½ lower R. S.		¼ gr. of antimony every two hours; blisters applied; afterwards diuretics.	A weakly woman, allowed to linger too long in the hospital.	Vol. 18, p. 15.
105	C. M'Lean	16	Good	7	17	45	120, soft	?	½ lower R. S.		Antimony ¼ gr. and diuretics.	Detained in the hospital on account of pleurisy.	Vol. 19, p. 128.
106	M. M'Donald	40	Weak	2	6	21	120, full and strong	32 to 36, hurried	½ lower L. S.		Antimony ¼ gr. every third hour; afterwards diminished to ⅙ gr. every fourth hour; 8 *leeches.*	This patient was a night nurse, and suffered from debility and leucorrhœa.	Vol. 18, p. 150.

No.	Name.	Age.	Previous Health.	First seen after K'port. Days.	Convalescence after K'port. Days.	In Hospital. Days.	Pulse. Lowest recorded of Treat- ment.	Respiration. At commencement of Treatment.	Extent, and Side involved.	Complication.	Treatment.	Observations.—As to Nature of Case—Kind of Complication—Violence of Symptoms—Peculiarity of Physical Signs—Sequelæ, &c. &c.	Reference to Record of Hospital Case Books, Ward 11.
107	J. Gordon	58	Good	6	11	88	114, bounding	40, hur- ried	3 lower L. S.		4 gr. of antimony every hour; 10 leeches, and a blister; diuretics, treated with antifungals.	A robust woman, who recovered rapid ly, but, per luxurism, remained in the house for two months after convalescence.	Vol. 20, p. 2
108	J. Jackson	34	Not good	6	14	19	96, not along	Dys- pnœa	4 upper R. S.	×	Salines; expectorants; nutrients.	Cough and expectoration for 13 years, with occasional hæmoptysis.	Vol. 21, p. 27.
109	I. Douglas D 27	42	Not good	1	15	61	96, soft and pulsat- ing	53, la- boured	4 lower L. S. 4 lower R. S. D.	×	The acute rheumatism and pericarditis which existed throughout this case were treated with alkalies and diuretics; the pneumonia with blisters, stimulants, and nutrients.	This was a case of acute rheumatism and heart disease. The pneumonia ran its course in 15 days.	Vol. 25, p. 38.
110	M. Armstrong	38	Strong	1	7	12	105, com- pressible	24, easy	4 lower R. S.	×	Wine ℥vj and nutrients.	Supervened on severe erysipelas of the face, 3 days after admission.	Vol. 25, p. 111.
111	A. Mackay D 23	43	Weak	11	12	24	130, weak	Urgent dys- pnœa	4 lower R. S., 4 mid- dle L. S.	×	Wine ℥vj; nutrients?	Subject to cough for three years pre- viously.	Vol. 26, p. 82.
112	B. Dickson Unc. s.	36	Bad	2	4	8	85, weak	Dys- pnœa	4 lower R. S.	×	Diuretics; blister applied; wine ℥iv.	Complicated with albuminuria and delirium.	Vol. 20, p. 64.
113	M. Drummond D 29	39	Good	5	10	19	86, weak	30, dys- pnœal	4 lower L. S., 4 lower R. S.		Nutrients; wine ℥iijss.	Little fever. Slight pneumonia on the left side, which soon disappeared. Dense hepatisation on right side.	Vol. 20, p. 290.
114	J. Dunlop	17	Bad	1	9	19	130, weak	Dys- pnœa	4 lower R. S.	×	Salines; nutrients; wine ℥iv.	Complicated with bronchitis and pericarditis.	Vol. 35, p. 94.
115	S. Hardin	17	Good	7	15	17	86, weak	Dys- pnœa	Whole of L. S.		Salines with nitric ether; ℥j of wine every two hours, and strong beef-tea ℥iii.	Very weak on admission.	Vol. 33, p. 29.
116	R. Clarke D 38	18	Cough for a twelve- month	2	14	21	104, small	56, ur- gent dys- pnœa	4 lower L. R. S., 4 upper R. S.		At first salines; afterwards diuretics; ℥j of wine every half hour; now milk and strong beef-tea ad lib.	The double pneumonia proved an un- favourable case. Great weakness and dyspnœa. Faced by ℥ss of wine every half hour.	Vol. 34, p. 36.
117	G. Robertson	70	Bronchitis	5	14	42	100, small and weak	Dys- pnœa	4 bases R. S.	×	Expectorants; wine ℥vj; nutrients.	Complicated with mitral incompe- tence and bronchitis.	Vol. 33, p. 20.

118	A. White	35	Weak	6	11	49	115, fair strength.	36	Whole of R. S.		Salines; wine ℥iij, and steak diet.	Pneumonia over whole of right side all disappeared. Afterwards tubercular condensation of right apex.	Vol. 36, p. 33.
119	A. English	35	Good	7	12	73	102, feeble	Orthopnœa	¼ lower R. S.	X	Salines; beef-tea, wine ℥vj.	Preceded by abortion, and accompanied by bronchitis and phthisis.	Vol. 38, p. 230.
120	A. Kinniburgh	19	Long cough	8	16	23	108, feeble	Orthopnœa	¾ lower R. S.	X	Beef-tea; wine ℥iv.	Had cough for 17 years following measles. Pleurisy.	Vol. 38, p. 215.
121	E. Bruce	27	Long cough	7	18	60	98, feeble	†	⅕ lower L. S.	X	Beef-tea; wine ℥iv.	Long had cough. Phthisis. Pleurisy.	Vol. 40, p. 118.
122	A. Aitken	17	Good	3	11	13	116, moderate	36, tranquil	¼ lower R. S.	X	Beef-tea; wine ℥vj.	Complicated with pleurisy.	Vol. 44, p. 68.
123	E. Ainslie	37	Good	4	11	19	106, weak	28	¼ lower R. S.		Beef-tea; wine ℥iv.	A simple pneumonia.	Vol. 44, p. 118.
124	Jessie Baxter	56	Good	5	17	16	120, weak	66, dyspnœa	Whole R. S.		Salines; wine ℥iv; nutrients.	Treated previously for an abscess in the axilla.	Vol. 42, p. 168.
125	C. M'Pherson	46	Good	8	23	21	108, soft, weak	35, dyspnœa	Whole R. S.		Wine ℥iv ad ℥vj; nutrients; salines, with vin. colchici.	A healthy woman, but very weak on admission.	Vol. 48, p. 1.

FATAL COMPLICATED CASES.

No.	Name.	Age	Extent, and Side Involved.	COMPLICATION CAUSING DEATH.	Reference to Record in Hospital Case Books.
126	T. Morrison	18	¼ upper R. S.	Had uncontrollable diarrhœa from the first, apparently excited by purgatives before admission. He sank exhausted in five days, notwithstanding the use of astringents, opiates, nutrients, and latterly stimulants. On dissection, in addition to hepatization of lung, enlargement and extensive ulceration of follicles in jejunum and ilium.	Vol. 31, p. 73. Ward 1.
127	Margt. Currie	37	½ lower R. S.	This woman had albuminuria, and was first attacked with headache and vomiting. She entered the house on the 8th day of the pneumonia, when delirium came on, and died the day after admission. No examination of the body could be obtained.	Vol. 1, p. 159. Ward 11.
128	D. Murray	48	⅓ lower R. S.	Two days after admission the mind became confused, and he died delirious 3 days subsequently of acute meningitis.	Vol. 16, p. 37. Ward 1.
129	Margt. Lamont	40	Whole of R. S.	She was recovering from the pneumonia when, on the 13th day, fatal meningitis appeared. She had also aneurism of an aortic valve.	Case book missing.

With regard to treatment, it will be observed that the
earlier cases were ordered larger doses of tartar emetic than
the later ones, and that in the last cases this drug [was not
prescribed at all. By *Salines* is to be understood small doses
of the acetate of ammonia, with $\frac{1}{4}$ of a grain of tartar emetic.
By *Diuretics* is to be understood ℥j doses of Sp. Æther. Nit.,
sometimes associated with ℥x of Tr. Vin. Sem. Colchici.
By *Nutrients* is to be understood bea-tea and milk, taken
early, with beef-steaks, mutton-chops, and eggs, as soon as
they could be eaten by the patient. In the first cases, it will
be seen they accompanied other treatment, and though not
specially mentioned, were still given. In the latest cases
they constituted the whole treatment.

Concerning the mortality connected with pneumonia, it
is necessary to observe, that in addition to the four fatal cases
recorded, I have found in the pathological registers kept by
Drs. Gairdner, Haldane, and Grainger Stewart, thirteen other
cases, in which as the result of chronic, cerebral, spinal, cardiac, hepatic, renal, or other pulmonary disease (such as
phthisis and chronic bronchitis), pneumonia appeared before
death, adding a fatal complication to previously existing
maladies. Not one of these c..n properly be considered as a
case of acute or primary pneumonia. They have all been
entered by the clerks in the ward-books as softening of the
brain or spinal cord, morbus cordis, phthisis, Bright's disease,
cirrhosis of the liver, or other lesion, for which the patients
entered the Infirmary and were treated. In most of them it
was the *pneumonie des agonizans* of the French, and in all
must be regarded as the consecutive chronic or latent pneumonias of medical writers.

These, then, are positively all the cases of acute pneumonia which have entered the clinical wards of the Infirmary,
when under my care, during the last sixteen years, so far as
I can discover them. Every case has been treated publicly,

and is open for inspection in the ward-books; and the result is that the mortality of all the acute pneumonias, complicated and uncomplicated, in the practice of the clinical wards while under my care, is, up to February 1865, 1 death in 32½ cases. Taking only the cases of uncomplicated pneumonia, however, 105 in number, not one has died, although many of them have been very severe, involving the whole of one lung in 15, and portions of both lungs in 26 cases.

In the four fatal cases, death was evidently caused by complications independent of the pneumonia. They ought to be regarded as pathological accidents, for in not one of them could the pulmonary disease be properly regarded even as assisting the mortality. The Table shows that in many instances where weakness was much greater than existed in any of them, pneumonia rapidly passed through its natural progress. To arrive at true statistics *with regard to treatment*, therefore, it becomes necessary to eliminate these four cases, as has been done by many other hospital physicians, and to fix our attention on the first 125 cases reported in the previous table.

Sex.—Of these 125 cases, 85 were males and 40 were females. In the Table, the latter have been enumerated after, and so separated from the former.

Age.—The average of the males was 31½ years; the average age of the females, 28¼ years; the average age of both 30½ years. Between the ages of 5 and 15 years was 1 case—a girl; between 10 and 20 years, 29 cases—12 females; between 20 and 30 years, 35 cases—11 females; between 30 and 40 years, 23 cases—7 females; between 40 and 50 years, 24 cases—5 females; between 50 and 60 years, 11 cases—1 female; between 60 and 70 years, 1 case—a female; and between 70 and 80 years, 1 case—a female.

The state of health previous to the attack of pneumonia was recorded in 118 cases. Of these 84 were males and 34 were females, and we have to determine the influence exercised by the general health—1st, On the duration of the disease; and 2dly, On the duration of the convalescence.

Of the 84 males, 57 were in good, and 27 in impaired health. The average duration of the disease in the former was 12 days and in the latter 16½ days. Of the 34 females, 12 only were in good, and 22 were in impaired health. The average duration of the disease in the former was 14 days, and in the latter 16 days.

In determining the influence of health on the convalescence, it becomes necessary to deduct from the 57 male cases those which remained in the house in consequence of severe complications, want of clothes, or other causes unconnected with the pneumonia. These were 10 in number. Among the 47 which remain, several, though marked as having good health previous to the occurrence of the disease, were still in a state of great exhaustion on entering the Infirmary, either from previous bleeding or starvation. The average duration of the convalescence, including such cases, was 15½ days. For the same reason, deducting 5 from the 28 cases which are described as weak on admission, or who had had cough, rheumatism, or other weakening disease previous to the pneumonia, the average duration of convalescence in the remaining 23 cases was 23½ days. Of the 34 women, the average duration of the convalescence in the 12 recorded as being previously in good health was 14 days. Of the 22 females said to have impaired health previous to the attack of pneumonia—after deducting 6 whose residence was prolonged by complications—the average duration of the 16 which remain was 23¾ days.

Simple or uncomplicated Pneumonia.—Of the 125 cases

there were 105 simple or uncomplicated, and 20 complicated.
Of the former there were 74 males and 31 females. 79 were
single and 26 double cases. Of these I find that the clerk
has omitted to state either the exact day of rigor or of convalescence in six, so that no conclusion can be derived from
them as to the duration of the disease. Of the remaining 99
cases, 73 were single, and 26 double, and the duration of the
disease in the whole on an average, was 14¼ days.

*The duration of the disease in the 73 cases of single uncom-
plicated pneumonia*, counting from the occurrence of rigor to
the commencement of convalescence, was as follows :—2 cases
recovered in 5 days ; 4 cases in 7 days ; 5 cases in 8 days ;
2 cases in 9 days ; 8 cases in 10 days ; 7 cases in 11 days ;
7 cases in 12 days ; 4 cases in 13 days ; 13 cases in 14 days ;
2 cases in 15 days ; 3 cases in 16 days ; 3 cases in 17 days ;
3 cases in 18 days ; 1 case in 19 days ; 2 cases in 20 days ;
8 cases in 21 days ; 1 case in 22 days ; 2 cases in 23 days ;
and 1 case in 26 days. The average duration 13⅞ days.

*The duration of the disease in the 26 cases of double uncom-
plicated pneumonia*, counting from the occurrence of the rigor
to the commencement of convalescence, was as follows :—2
cases recovered in 8 days ; 1 case in 9 days ; 2 cases in 10
days ; 2 cases in 11 days ; 1 case in 12 days ; 1 case in 13
days ; 4 cases in 14 days ; 1 case in 15 days ; 2 cases in 16
days ; 2 cases in 18 days ; 2 cases in 19 days ; 1 case in 20
days ; 3 cases in 21 days ; 1 case in 27 days ; 1 case in 55
days. The average duration 16⅘ days.*

Effects of bleeding.—Of the 105 simple or uncomplicated
cases there were 9 bled by venesection, and subjected to an

---

* If the case of Hogg (No. 6), a weak young man, much reduced by bleeding and other antiphlogistic treatment before admission, and the duration of
whose disease in consequence was 55 days, be subtracted, the average duration
of these double cases would only be 14 days.

antiphlogistic treatment, before or immediately upon admission, before I saw them. The amount of blood extracted varied from 12 to 30 oz., the latter in two bleedings. The duration of one case is not stated. Of the remaining 8 cases, the duration was as follows :—One case recovered in 7 days ; 2 cases in 14 days ; 1 case in 16 days ; 1 case in 17 days ; 1 case in 20 days ; 1 case in 27 days ; and 1 case in 55 days. The average duration was $21\frac{1}{4}$ days.

In addition to the 9 cases bled by venesection, there were 16 others who were cupped, or had a few leeches applied, for the most part as a palliative. It did not occur to me that such cases would have been referred to as illustrative of the effects of bleeding in pneumonia ; but as these have been ingeniously added by a critic to the 9 previous cases, and represented as 25 of my cases which were bled, constituting 20 per cent of the whole number,* it becomes necessary to ascertain the facts they present. Two of these cases could not tell to what extent they had lost blood by cupping (cases 72 and 74), and in 2 cases the day of convalescence was not determined (cases 72 and 91). In the other cases the amount of blood lost, and the day of convalescence, were as follows, allowing $\frac{1}{2}$ oz. of blood lost for each leech applied :— One case lost $1\frac{1}{2}$ oz. of blood, and recovered in 21 days ; 6 cases lost 4 oz. of blood ; and subtracting 1 in whom the convalescence was not determined, the 5 others recovered, on an average, in 10 days ; 1 case lost 5 oz. of blood, and recovered in 11 days ; 1 case lost $5\frac{1}{4}$ oz. from two applications of leeches (case 102), and recovered in 26 days ; 4 cases lost 6 oz. of blood, and recovered, on an average, in 23 days ; and 1 case lost 8 oz. of blood, and recovered in 14 days. The average duration of the disease in the 14 cases thus bled by cupping and leeching, in whom the day of recovery was ascertained, was $15\frac{4}{14}$.

* See Brit. Med. Journ., November 18, 1865, p. 532.

The duration of residence in hospital of the single uncomplicated cases of pneumonia—excluding 2 cases in which the date of dismission is omitted, making 77 cases—was on the average, 21¾ days. For the males (52) 18⅔ days, and for the females (25) 27½ days. Of the 26 double uncomplicated cases, the average duration of residence in hospital was 23¾ days. Of the males (20) 23¹⅓₀ days; of the females (6) 22⅔ days.

All these averages are far too high, as will be at once seen on referring to the Column of Observations in the Table, Nos. 14, 17, 18, 19, 27, 29, 50, 51, 100, 104, 105, 107, 109, in all which, detention in the house, for various reasons irrespective of the pneumonia, makes the period of residence on account of that disease much too long.

The average duration of residence in hospital of 8 cases, bled early in the disease by venesection (the 9th case being excluded in consequence of the day of dismission not being entered in the case-book), was 32 days.

The extent of pulmonary tissue involved in the pneumonia was carefully determined by percussion and auscultation from the amount of dulness, crepitation, tubular breathing, and increased vocal resonance present in each case. The average duration of the disease in the 95 single cases remaining after deduction of the 10 unsatisfactory ones, counting from the rigor to the commencement of convalescence, was as follows : —⅙ of the lung (2 cases), average duration, 8½ days ; ⅓ the lung (12 cases), 12 days ; ½ the lung (25 cases), 15¾ days ; ⅔ the lung (34 cases), 14 days ; ¾ the lung (6 cases), 14⅓ days ; ⅘ the lung (1 case) 12 days ; the whole lung (15 cases), 10½ days. Of these 95 cases, the right lung was affected in 58, the left lung in 37.

Pneumonia confined to the upper lobe occurred among the

95 single cases in 11, or nearly 1 in 9 of the whole, and the average duration of the disease in these was 13 days, and of their residence in the hospital 14½ days.

Complicated cases of Pneumonia.—Of the 20 complicated cases of pneumonia, 16 were single and 4 double, and the duration of the disease on an average was 15½ days.

Of the 16 single complicated cases, the duration of the disease cannot be determined in 3. Of the remaining 13, the duration was as follows :—One case recovered in 7 days ; 2 cases in 9 days ; 1 case in 10 days ; 1 case in 12 days ; 2 cases in 14 days ; 1 case in 15 days ; 2 cases in 16 days ; 2 cases in 19 days ; and 1 case in 48 days. The average duration, 16 days.

Of the 4 double cases of complicated pneumonia, 1 case recovered in 9 days ; 1 case in 14 days ; 1 case in 15 days ; and one case in 18 days. The average duration 14 days.

A careful study of the preceding facts will, I think, tend to establish some new truths, and correct several prevailing errors with regard to pneumonia. I would remind those, however, who, being yet sceptical as to the value of a restorative treatment, may imagine that some of these cases might not have been pneumonia, that they were all diagnosed, and treated publicly in the Royal Infirmary ; were examined not only by myself, but by my intelligent clerks and assistants, and were all made the subject of Clinical Lectures and commentaries at the bedside. In all of them the physical signs and the functional symptoms were precisely and minutely recorded. There is, therefore, the positive certainty not only that every one of these cases was a genuine example of pneumonia, but that no other cases of the disease but what are tabulated were treated by me during the period referred to. It should be explained, however, that a few cases were partly treated by my colleagues either before I assumed duty, or after I left it, in the too frequent changes which occur among the Clinical Professors in this University. Such cases are not inserted. It is also necessary to point out that two or three cases brought into the house by the police in an exhausted condition, and who died before I saw them, are not inserted. It is the more important to refer to such occurrences, because they serve to account for the differences which must always exist between the general hospital and clinical statistics. Grisolle has very unjustly alluded to this difference in the hospital of Vienna, with a view of throwing distrust on the conclusions of Dietl. (2d edit. pp. 564, 565.) But every hospital physician must be aware that the records of the dead-room, or of the hospital generally, afford no index whatever to the number of acute pneumonias treated clinically, comprehending as they do not only consecutive, latent, and chronic pneumonias, but not unfrequently cases of pneumonia which have entered the house in a dying condition, and have not been treated at all.

1. The first great fact which the preceding figures serve to establish is, that simple primary pneumonia, whether single or double, if treated by the restorative plan, is not a fatal disease. Surely 105 consecutive cases, of which 26 were double, are sufficient to establish this proposition, especially when it is considered that they were diffused over sixteen years, and occurred in all seasons. Among these, also, the whole of one lung was involved in no less than 15 cases, and the symptoms in many of them were exceedingly severe. Neither will anything that has been said as to strength of constitution, or change of type in disease, explain the result, as several of the cases were those of healthy vigorous young labourers, whilst others were those of weak and broken down sempstresses. In any and every case the disease goes through its natural progress, if the system be not too much exhausted, either naturally or by the inter-

ference of the physician ; and if a judicious restorative treatment be adopted.

2. As a general rule, it will be observed that prostration and weakening complications or remedies not only lengthen the period of the disease, but especially prolong the convalescence. This will be seen on referring to Nos. 6, 20, 71, 100, 101, 104, 118, and 119 in the Table. An analysis of the whole number of cases shows that women, even when in good health, recover less quickly than men ; and that when the health is impaired in both sexes, the difference in the duration of the disease and of the convalescence is strongly marked—especially in men. Thus, on the average, the disease lasts 8½ days longer in a weak man than in a strong one, while the period of convalescence is 8½ days longer. Among the women, weak individuals were more numerous than healthy ones, and in them the disease lasted 2 days, and the convalescence 9½ days longer on the average.

3. It is generally supposed that the amount of lung affected by pneumonia must influence the result and duration of the disease. As to the result, all my cases recovered, even the 15 cases where the whole of one lung was involved, as well as the 26 cases where portions of both lungs were affected. In one complicated case (No. 66) the whole lung on the right side, and two-thirds of the lung on the left side were simultaneously involved, thus leaving only one-third of a lung to respire with, and yet without bleeding, but aided by nutrients and restoratives, the man was convalescent on the fourteenth day, and left the house quite well, after a sixteen days' residence. With regard to duration, the extent of the disease does not exert so much influence as is generally supposed. If only a fourth of one lung be affected, the recovery may take place in 8 days : but after that, whether the half or the whole of one lung, or two-thirds of both lungs, be involved, it does not appear to cause much difference. Cases

with half a lung pneumonic, recovered in 15, with two-thirds of a lung in 14, with a whole lung in 10, and with portions of both lungs in 14 days, on the average.

4. Since the observations of Louis, it has been supposed that a pneumonia at the apex of a lung was more fatal and more prolonged than one at the base; and so it may be with an antiphlogistic treatment. But with a restorative treatment, the preceding facts show that in 11 cases where the disease was confined to the apex, recovery took place in all, and on an average on the thirteenth day.

5. In no single instance has a case of acute pneumonia in my hands degenerated into the chronic form, or become gangrenous, even in the 11 cases where the disease was confined to the apex. Several cases, however, have entered the house already chronic from neglect, want of nutrients, or as the result of a lowering treatment—circumstances that indicate sufficiently well the causes which produce it.

6. Among the whole number of my cases, deaths only occurred from severe complications, a circumstance which induces me to believe that under a restorative treatment, begun early in the case, the influence of age and sex on the mortality is not appreciable. Neither is the duration of the disease much influenced by complication so long as the general health is not impaired.

7. Although among the few cases bled by venesection there is sufficient evidence to prove that the practice prolonged convalescence in the weak and was useless in the strong (see Appendix, cases III. VI and VIII), no conclusion can be derived from my cases as to the results of limited bleedings (from 3 to 8 oz), either as to their influence on the progress of the disease, or their utility even as palliatives.

COMPARATIVE STATISTICS AS TO THE TREATMENT OF ACUTE PNEUMONIA.

In order that the contrast between my own cases and those of other practitioners may be as exact and fair as possible, I propose only to refer to such as are drawn from a pretty equal or a larger number of cases. For the same reason, I shall not jumble the experiences of different practitioners together under one head, or confound the statistics of a whole general hospital with those of an individual practitioner in it. I shall, in the first place, condense shortly the results of each; then give the general hospital statistics of pneumonia; and lastly, contrast the whole with the results of my own practice.

I. *Results of Bleeding in Pneumonia.*—The total number of cases, recorded by M. Louis, was 107.[*] Of these 32 died, or 1 in 3⅓. In 78 of those cases, which occurred at La Charité, bleeding was performed from the first to the ninth day, and the deaths were 28, or 1 in 3⅓. The duration of the disease in the cases which recovered was 15½ days. Of the remaining 29 cases, which occurred at La Pitié, the bleeding was performed earlier, that is during the first 4 days, and of these only 4 died, that is 1 in 7½. The duration of the disease, however, in the cases that recovered, was 18⅓ days. This diminished mortality, but greater length of recovery, M. Louis attributes to the bleedings not having been so large, and the greater amount of tartar emetic employed. Hence, the proposition he sought to establish, that although bleeding has a very limited influence on pneumonia, it should be practised early. With regard to M. Louis's results, it should be remembered, 1st, That the cases which were unfavourable from previous bad health, or from other causes, were excluded, so that all his patients enjoyed excellent health when they were

* Recherches sur les effets de la Saignée. Paris, 1835.

attacked; 2dly, That they were uncomplicated, and that the duration of the disease was estimated from the occurrence of febrile symptoms, up to the time when light food could be taken, which was generally three days after the fever had ceased.

II. M. Bouillaud's[*] account of his treatment by the *coup sur coup* treatment is, that of 102 cases treated by him from 1831 to 1834, the deaths were 12—that is, 1 death in 8½ cases.

III. In a memoir by M. Briquet[†] there is some confusion of numbers. He informs us that his cases were 141 (T. 7, p. 477), but in giving the ages of these, he enumerates 144 cases (T. 7, p 479); and in speaking of the influence of age on mortality, his cases are only 140 (T. 9, p. 28). Of these 140 cases, 29 died; that is, there was a mortality of more than 1 death in 5 cases. Almost all these cases were bled, according to the strength of the patient (T. 8, p. 283). In three-fourths of the cases, blisters and tartar emetic were also employed.

IV. M. Grisolle[‡] advocated more moderate bleedings than those so frequently had recourse to, his conscience preventing the abandonment of venesection altogether (p. 561). He analyses 75 cases of Bouillaud, pointing out that only 49 were treated by the *coup-sur-coup* mode of bleeding, of which 6 died, or 1 in 8 cases, a favourable result, which he attributes to the youth of the patients treated. Of his own cases, one group of 50 cases were bled only in the first stage of the disease; of these 5 died, or 1 in 10. Those cases that died were bled most, each losing about 4 lb. 4 oz. of blood in successive bleedings. All the cases in this group were uncomplicated, and of the average age of 40 years. Of the 45 who recovered, convalescence commenced on the 10th day, and they resumed their occupations on the 21st day, as an average. Of 182 cases that were bled in the second stage, 32 died, or more than 1 in 6. Here also those who died

* Art. Pneumonie, Dict. de Médicine, en 15 vol., 1835.
† Archiv. Gen. de Médicine, 3 Serie, Tom. 7, 8, 9. 1840.
‡ Traité pratique de la Pneumonie. Paris, 1841.

were bled most—the bleedings varying in amount from 8 or
12 oz. to 3 lbs. The average quantity lost was 3 lbs. All
the cases in this group were uncomplicated, and of the
average age of 35 years. Of the 150 cases that recovered,
convalescence commenced on the 17th day, and they resumed
their occupations on the 22d day—as an average. He admits
that the pneumonia can never be jugulated by bleeding. Of
the whole 232 cases, 37 died—that is, about 1 in 6½—as the
general result of M. Grisolle's hospital practice, a mortality
only one-half that of M. Louis's cases, although the circumstances under which they occurred were the same, with the
exception of not being so heroically treated. Laennec also,
who only bled moderately at the commencement of the
disease, regarded the mortality to be 1 death in 6 or 8 cases.*

In 1864 M. Grisolle published another edition of his work,
in which these same statistics are repeated without any
change whatever, and this notwithstanding his acquaintance
with the author's researches, and the immense improvements
which have taken place in the art and science of medicine
during the long interval of 23 years. What seems very sur-
prising is, that he wishes to have it believed that his antiphlogistic treatment, with a mortality of 1 in 6 cases, is still the best.

V. Acerbi† bled largely and frequently in 142 cases, of
whom 16 died, or 1 in 9. Of those who died 4 had been bled
from three to four times; 5 from five to eight times; and
7 from nine to thirteen times. 30 of the 142 were bled from
ten to twenty times, 12 ounces each time, who therefore lost
from 120 to 240 ounces. From 4 to 8 grains of tartar emetic
were also given daily.

VI. Dietl treated 85 cases by large bleedings, of whom 17
died, that is 1 in 5.

VII. In 1842 Dr. Hughes* published an account of 101 cases treated for the most part antiphlogistically in Guy's Hospital, of whom 24 died, or 1 in 4½. Of those, however, only 47 were actively treated by bleeding, antimony, calomel and opium, etc. In 37, general bleeding was not practised. The complications, excluding pleurisy and bronchitis, were 27, and the double cases 19.

VIII. The most successful account of the treatment of pneumonia by bleeding is that published by Wossidlo,† who treated 112 cases, of whom 4 died, or 1 death in 28 cases. There were only 11 complications, including 4 with tubercle, 2 with blenorrhœa, 1 with catarrh, 2 with pregnancy, 1 with sciatica, and 1 with atrophia mesenterica. 50 of his cases, however, were below 20 years of age; and 44 of these were children below 10 years of age. To these it seems only a few leeches were applied. The amount to which he bled, and the diet given to the adults, are not stated.

IX. Dr. Glen, my former resident clerk, was so good as to tabulate for me all the cases of pneumonia given in the army returns, and reported by Colonel Tulloch.‡ These returns give us no information as to the mode in which the diagnosis was determined, or what was the treatment. The favourable mortality of 1 death in 13 cases, which, according to Dr. Glen, is the general result, is supposed to result from the bleedings having been performed early, and in young vigorous subjects.

X. *Treatment by large doses of Tartar Emetic.*—Rasori,§ in the great hospital of Milan, treated 648 cases by large doses

* Guy's Hospital Reports, vol. vii.
† Schmidt's Jahrbücher Band, Bd. 51, 1846, p. 125; and Brit. and For. Med. Chir. Review, July 1855, p. 16.
‡ Government Statistical Reports on Mortality among the Troops. 1853.
§ From an analysis of Rasori's practice—Annales de Thérapeutique, Janvier 1847.

of tartar emetic, of which 555 were cured, and 143 died, that is, 1 in 4½. In publishing this statement, Rasori gives the result as one more favourable than the practice of bloodletting, which of course he would not have done unless the latter treatment was then well known to have been attended with a greater mortality than that by tartar emetic, or 1 death in 4½ cases.

XI. M. Grisolle treated 154 cases with large doses of tartar emetic, of which 29 died—that is, 1 in 5½; and (XII.) Dietl treated 106 cases, of which 22 died—that is, little more than 1 in 5.

XIII. Von Wahl treated, during six years in St. Petersburg, 354 cases, of whom 84 died, or 1 in 4⅔ cases.* Only those having great congestion were bled, but in most cases tartar emetic was given in large doses early. (XIV.) Thielmann,† in the Peter and Paul's Hospital of St. Petersburg, treated with large doses of tartar emetic 110 cases of pneumonia, of which 12 died, or 1 in 9⅓. Opium was given to check diarrhœa.

Expectant or Dietetic Treatment.—This treatment essentially consists in allowing the disease to go through its natural course. During the stage of fever diet is light, or withheld altogether, and cold water allowed for drink; subsequently better diet is allowed, and occasionally wine, according to the nature of the symptoms. Sometimes a dietetic is converted into an *expectant treatment*, when remedies are given to meet occasional symptoms, as in the practice of Skoda, in the Charity Hospital of Vienna (XV.) An account of this has been given to us by Dr. George Balfour, who found from the books of the hospital, that during a period of three years and five months, commencing 1843, 392 patients were treated, of whom 54 died, or 1 in 7¼. Occasionally opium was given in small doses if there was much pain. Venesection was also

---

* Petersburg Med. Zeit., i. 6, 1801. Canstatt, 1851, p. 237.
† Canstatt, 1852; iii. p. 231.

practised early if there was much dyspnœa, and emetics given if the expectoration consisted of tough mucus.

Dr. G. Balfour has also given some statistics of the Homœopathic Hospital of Vienna, but accompanied with statements which render it doubtful whether every case that applied was admitted, and consequently not fairly comparable with other hospital statistics. There can be no doubt, however, that many severe cases of pneumonia recovered under a system of treatment which, it appears to me, most medical men must consider to be essentially a dietetic one. The best homœopathic statistics are those of Tessier,* who had 3 deaths in 41 cases ; and (XVI.) of Wurmb of Vienna,† who of 119 cases had 8 deaths—nearly 1 in 15.

XVII. Dr. Diatl published in 1848 an account of 189 cases treated by diet only, of which 14 died, that is 1 in 13½. The following is his table of 380 cases, exhibiting the result of the three kinds of treatment :—

	Vene-section.	Tartar Emetic.	Diet.
Cured	68	84	175
Died	17	22	14
	85	106	189
Per cent	20.4	20.7	7.4
Deaths	1 in 5	1 in 5.22	1 in 13¼

It was further observable that of the 85 cases treated by blood-letting, 7 of the fatal cases were uncomplicated ; whilst of the 189 cases treated by diet, not one of the deaths was an uncomplicated one. In 1852 he gave the result of 750 cases, treated dietetically, of which 69 died, or 1 in 10.9.

We are informed by Grisolle (2me. edit., p. 570) that Legendre, after having treated the pneumonia of infants entirely by bleeding and antiphlogistics, left a memoir which

* Homœopathic Treatment of Pneumonia, 8vo, New York, 1855.
† Brit. Journal of Homœopathy, vol. iv. p. 75.

was published after his death,* in which he sought to show
that a dietetic treatment was far preferable. His views, which
were founded on only 15 cases, have since been supported by
(XVIII) M. Barthez, who, on the 8th of April 1862, informed
the Imperial Academy of Medicine, that of 212 children, varying in age from 2 to 15 years, he had treated in the hospital
of St. Eugenie, only 2 had died. Of these, however, what is
called a slightly active treatment was employed in ¼th of the
cases. In accepting this important result M. Grisolle only
sees in it a confirmation of the fact that pneumonia in young
subjects has a tendency to spontaneous recovery, but denies
that such treatment is useful at a more advanced age.

Mixed Treatment.—In recent times cases of pneumonia
have been treated after a mixed fashion, according to the
nature of the symptoms, but with no very marked beneficial
effect. As examples of this system I may refer to the
results given by Lebert, Huss, Bamberger, Flint, Rigler and
Morehead.

XIX. Deducting from the 222 pneumonic cases of Lebert† 17
which died on the day of entrance into the Zurich Hospital, or
on the following day, there remain 205, which he treated during
5 years, of whom 15 died—that is, exactly 1 death in 13⅔ cases.
4 cases were complicated, all of which died. The other 201
uncomplicated cases were regularly treated, and of these 11
died, or 1 in 18. Among the whole number were 22 double
cases. The treatment consisted of general and local bleeding
in the majority of the cases, but if there was prostration,
antimony in full doses was relied on. Various other remedies
were employed to meet particular indications, such as mercurial inunction, muriate of ammonia, acetate of lead, opium,
quinine, camphor, benzoin, etc. In the later stages with
weakness, he gave stimulants, nourishment, and wine.

* Archiv. Gen. de Médecins, September 1859.
† Handbuch der praktischen Medicin, Band 11, p. 69, 1859.

XX. The most important memoir recently published is that of Professor Huss of Stockholm,* who employed bleeding and heroic remedies in the early stage, and in the later ones antimony, mercury, and various remedies—among the rest turpentine, camphor, morphia, and quinine. During 16 years the number of cases treated was 2616, of which 281 died; that is 1 in 9½ cases. The uncomplicated cases were 1657, of whom 96 died, or 1 in 17 cases. The complicated cases were 959, of whom 185 died, or 1 in 5 cases. There were 384 cases of double pneumonia, of whom 88 died, rather more than 1 in 4½ cases. The treatment employed was adapted, as it was thought, to the emergencies of the case, and may be called a modified antiphlogistic practice, many cases not having been bled at all. Its superiority over the rigid antiphlogistic system, and even over that of Grisolle, therefore, is marked.

It was during the first 8 years that blood-letting, general and local, was practised. Of 1040 then treated, 120 died, or 1 in 9 cases; while during the second 8 years 1576 cases were treated, of whom 161 died, not quite 1 in 10 cases. This difference is not great, but still leads Huss to the conclusion that blood-letting is injurious to a curative result (p. 158). He found also that it prolonged the disease 3 days (p. 160). In the first two stages a low diet only was allowed.

XXI. Dr. Bamberger† treated 186 cases without general blood-letting in the Julius Hospital of Wurzburg. Only a few leeches and fomentations were applied in some cases, and inf. digitalis given internally, which he says so clearly diminished the temperature and lessened the pulse, as to constitute it an important remedy in fever. To assist expectoration, tartar emetic, kermes, mineral, ipecacuanha, and sal ammoniac,

* Die Behandlung der Lungen-entzundung, etc. Leipsig, 1861.
† Wiener Wochenschrift, No. 50, 1857; and Canstatts Jahresbericht, 1858, iii. p. 284.

were given in small doses. Occasionally emetics were administered, and narcotics to relieve restlessness and procure sleep. In the more adynamic forms, senega, arnica, benzoin, vin. antim., quinine, camphor, musk, and other remedies were prescribed. Nothing is said of diet or wine, nor of complicated cases. Of these cases, 21 died, or 1 in 9.

XXII. Dr. Flint[*] has given the result of 133 cases he treated, during 12 years, in the cities of New Orleans, Louisville, and Buffalo, in the United States of America, of whom 35 died —more than 1 in 4. Among the 112 uncomplicated cases were 19 deaths, and among the 21 complicated cases 16. There were 11 cases of double pneumonia, of which 8 died ; 37 cases where the whole right lung was involved, of which 19 died ; 9 cases where the whole left lobe was affected, of which 1 died ; that is of all the cases, 57, in which the pneumonia extended over two or more lobes, one-third died. Of the remaining uncomplicated cases only 2 died. The treatment varied according to the case ; 12 were bled, 12 were treated with tartar emetic ; 100 cases took opium in variable doses : of these 49 had full or large doses, among whom 11 died. Alcoholic stimulants and quinine were also occasionally employed.

XXIII. Rigler treated[†] in the General Hospital of Gratz 119 cases, of which 20 died, or 1 in 6 cases. Venesection was practised in only 4 cases—leeches were applied in several to remove local pain. A strictly dietetic regimen was enjoined to diminish fever, and if the pneumonia spread, tartar emetic to the extent of one grain a day was given. Demulcent mixtures, friction of the extremities, and morphia were also occasionally employed. The duration of the disease on the average was 21 days. Of the 119 cases, 14 were double; 16 had pleurisy ; 10 pericarditis ; 2 strong intestinal catarrh (diarrhœa ?), and 1 albuminuria.

* American Journal of the Med. Science. July 1852.
† Canstatt, 1858 ; iii. p. 235.

XXIV. During six years from 1848 to 1853, Dr. Morehead[*] treated in the Jamsetjee Jejeebhoy Hospital of Bombay 103 cases, of whom 32 died, or 1 in 3⅓ cases. The native Hindoos, we are told, are of feeble constitution. Only 3 therefore were bled generally, but local blood-letting was adopted in 57 cases. Tartar emetic, from a sixth to half a grain, every second, third, or fourth hour, was given in 66 cases; mercury in 21 cases; blisters in 52 cases, quinine, liquor potassæ, and stimulants were also given. Of the 71 cases which recovered, 14 were discharged within 10 days; 23 between 11 and 20 days; 16 between 21 and 30 days; 18 above 31 days. Nothing is said as to diet, but under the head of stimulants we are told these should be employed when the pulse fails, etc.

XXV. *Treatment by Iron and Copper.*—Kisself[†] of Eilenburg treated 112 cases of pneumonia, of whom 5 died with complications, or 1 death in 22 cases. Where the urine was alkaline, he gave an ounce of the tincture of acetate of iron daily; when it was acid, he gave one and a half drachms of the tincture of the acetate of copper daily. The duration of the disease was from 2 to 9 days; but when complicated with typhus phenomena, reached 16 days. The abstract in Canstatt does not inform us whether these cases were treated in a hospital, the nature of the complications, or the diet ordered.

XXVI. *Treatment by Stimulants.*—The late Dr. Todd[‡] abandoned the treatment of pneumonia by blood-letting and antiphlogistics about the same time that I did so myself, but was gradually led into a system of stimulation. He considered alcohol given in small but repeated doses as nutritive, and ordered half an ounce of brandy to be given every half hour, hour, or two hours, according to the urgency of the case. He also

* Clinical Researches of Disease in India, vol. ii. p. 315, et seq.
† Canstatt, 1852; iii. p. 229.   ‡ Clinical Lectures, by Beale, p. 310.

D

supported the patient by nutrients, and gave good beef-tea early. The result of this practice was, that among 53 cases he had 6 deaths, or about 1 in 9.

General Hospital Statistics.

It has already been stated that the general statistics of a public hospital afford no index to the number of cases of acute pneumonia treated clinically (p. 28). It must also be evident that in institutions which contain several physicians, who treat their cases in a different manner, little is to be learnt of that treatment by mixing their cases together. Hence the various General Hospital Statistics of pneumonia ought only to be compared with one another, and never referred to as a means of comparison with the individual practice of physicians.

Statistics of Pneumonia in the Royal Infirmary of Edinburgh.—My former clerk, Dr. Thorburn, was kind enough, at my request, to go over 208 case-books of the Infirmary, dated between the years 1812 and 1837, and belonging to twelve physicians, all of whom practised an antiphlogistic treatment. He found that of 103 cases of pneumonia, 55 were cured, 41 died, and 7 were relieved—that is, 1 death in 2¼ cases. Dr. Thorburn then carefully read over these 103 cases, and rejected all those that were incomplete, or which presented no evidence of having been pneumonia. The remainder were tabulated, and it may safely be said that they were all cases of pneumonia, or of acute inflammations of the chest closely allied to that disease, and the result was :—Number of cases, 50; died, 19; cured or relieved, 31—that is, more than 1 death in 3 cases. Since the 1st of July 1839 the cases of pneumonia have been regularly tabulated, with the following results, for which I am indebted to Mr. M'Dougall :—

CASES of PNEUMONIA treated in the Royal Infirmary, from 1st July 1839 to 1st October 1865, including Cases returned as Broncho-Pneumonia, Plouro-Pneumonia, and Broncho-Pleuro-Pneumonia.

Years.	Total No. of Cases entering the Infirmary.	Cases of Pneumonia.			Statistician.
		Total Treated.	Re-covered.	Died.	
1st July 1839 to 1st Oct. 1841	7,969*	139	90	49	Dr. John Reid.
1st Oct. 1841 to 1st Oct. 1842	5,537	42	26	16	Dr. T. Pea-
1st Oct. 1842 to 1st July 1843	2,760	41	26	15	cock.
1st July 1843 to 1st Oct. 1844	6,977*	31	20	11	
1st Oct. 1844 to 1st Oct. 1845	8,252	50	37	13	
„ 1845 „ 1846	3,638	67	51	16	Dr. Hughes Bennett.
„ 1846 „ 1847	7,435*	93	52	41	
„ 1847 „ 1848	7,064*	104	60	44	
„ 1848 „ 1849	3,630†	88	71	17	Mr. M'Dougall.
„ 1849 „ 1850	3,079	81	65	16	„
„ 1850 „ 1851	4,537	73	52	21	„
„ 1851 „ 1852	4,341	106	86	20	„
„ 1852 „ 1853	4,262	84	63	21	„
„ 1853 „ 1854	4,211	67	54	13	„
„ 1854 „ 1855	3,990	64	53	11	„
„ 1855 „ 1856	3,816	68	56	12	„
„ 1856 „ 1857	3,558‡	39	36	3	„
„ 1857 „ 1858	3,465	61	56	5	„
„ 1858 „ 1859	3,718	50	43	7	„
„ 1859 „ 1860	3,594	54	43	11	„
„ 1860 „ 1861	3,937	78	70	8	„
„ 1861 „ 1862	3,892	73	63	10	„
„ 1862 „ 1863	4,384	86	75	11	„
„ 1863 „ 1864	4,253	59	49	10	„
„ 1864 „ 1865	4,585	48	42	6	„

These cases naturally divide themselves into three periods. During the first of these, previous to 1848, the old anti-phlogistic practice was the rule in the Infirmary; and the result was that of 567 cases 205 died, or 1 death in 2¾ cases.

* At these periods there were great epidemics of fever

† At this period considerable changes took place among the medical staff of the Infirmary, and the author first commenced a restorative treatment.

‡ Now commenced the blood-letting controversy, which strongly drew attention to the advantage of a restorative treatment.

At the commencement of the second period, occupying a period of eight years, I entered on my duties as a Clinical Professor, and the treatment by non-bleeding and restoratives was openly taught and practised by myself; and the result was that of 631 cases 131 died, or rather less than 1 death in 4¾ cases.

It was at the beginning of the third period, in 1856-57, that the attention of the profession was strongly drawn to the subject of pneumonia by the discussions which took place between Dr. Alison, myself, and others, and the so-called blood-letting controversy took place. This period extends up to the present time—nine years—during which an antiphlogistic practice has been the exception, although some of the Infirmary physicians have given tartar emetic in tolerably full doses, others opium, and others calomel. The result is that of 548 cases only 71 died, or 1 death in 7¾ cases.

The last nine years' experience of the treatment of pneumonia in the Royal Infirmary of Edinburgh therefore exhibits a mortality of 1 death in 7¾; that which existed before 1848 having been 1 death in 2¾ cases. The result is striking, and proves that nearly three times as many persons now recover as did so formerly. Nor have I any doubts that when large doses of antimony, calomel, and opium, and a mixed treatment, are abandoned, and a vigorous restorative treatment becomes the rule, the mortality will be still further diminished. Even as it is, the foregoing figures contrast favourably with those of some other hospitals. For, according to Dr. Arthur Mitchell,[*] the number of cases of pneumonia admitted into the General Hospital of Vienna from 1847 to 1858 inclusive—that is, for 10 years—was 5909, of which 1439 died, or 1 death in 4·1 cases. Dr. Arnold von Franque[†] informs us that in sixteen years, from 1849 to 1855 inclusive, there were admitted into the Julius Hospital of Würzburg

---

[*] Edin. Med. Journ. vol. iii. p. 399.
[†] Inaugural Dissertation, Würzburg, 1856, p. 42.

874 cases of pneumonia, of which 176 died—nearly 1 death in 5 cases. These proportions have undergone very little change since, for we find that in the Wieden Hospital of Vienna, according to Dinstl,* during five years (1857 to 1861), among 33,557 cases, 1212 cases of pneumonia were treated, of whom 277 died, or 1 in 4½—considered by the reporter to be a favourable result. During a similar period of five years (1856 to 1860) in the General Hospital of the same city, 3014 cases of pneumonia were treated, of whom 748 died, or a little more than 1 in 4 cases.

Conclusions derived from the preceding statistical facts.

With a view of rendering the inquiry as exact as possible, I have omitted from the preceding list all experiences which are not on the same footing as my own with regard to extent and other circumstances, with the exception of the treatment by stimulants, and this because the statistics given by the late Dr. Todd are the only ones as yet published as to the effects of those remedies. For the same reason I have omitted the recent researches of Hannover, as to 1382 cases of chest inflammations,† not being able from the abstract in Canstatt to determine the exact mortality and treatment of pneumonia, as distinguished from other thoracic affections. Numerous other valuable papers have on the like ground not been referred to. I feel satisfied, however, from their perusal that they add nothing of essential importance to the facts which have been already recorded.

These, then, I think distinctly prove—

1. That an extreme antiphlogistic treatment has always been attended with a large mortality, amounting to 1 death in 3 cases; but that when modified in various ways—that is, by diminishing the amount of lowering remedies, selecting

* Canstatt, 1862. iii. p. 219.   † Ibid. iii. p.224, 1864.

cases, or by the cases being those of young and vigorous subjects—the mortality varies from 1 death in $4\frac{1}{4}$ (VII.*) to 1 death in 13 cases (IX.)

2. That when one-half the cases are those of children, or persons below twenty years of age, and the lowering treatment slight, the mortality diminishes to 1 death in 28 cases (VIII.)

3. That a treatment by large doses of tartar emetic has been accompanied by a mortality varying from 1 death in $4\frac{1}{4}$ (X.) to 1 death in $9\frac{1}{2}$ cases (XIV.)

4. That a dietetic or expectant treatment has been followed by a mortality varying from 1 death in $7\frac{1}{4}$ (XV.) to 1 death in 10·9 cases (XVII.) In children, according to Barthez (XVIII.) the mortality is almost *nil.*

5. That the results of a mixed treatment, in which various remedies have been employed, according to the nature of the case and the stage of the disease, are a mortality varying from 1 death in $3\frac{1}{2}$ (XXIV.) to 1 death in $13\frac{3}{4}$ cases (XIX.).

6. That a tonic treatment with iron and copper, according to Kissel, was attended with a mortality of 1 death in 22 cases (XXV.)

7. That a treatment by stimulants, according to Todd, was followed by a mortality of 1 death in 9 cases (XXVI.)

8. That the restorative treatment of the author having been attended, in the worst point of view, by a mortality of only 1 death in $32\frac{1}{2}$ cases, is the most satisfactory yet published. But when it is considered that the 4 deaths resulted from pathological complications unconnected with the pneumonia, this treatment may be said to render the mortality in true cases of pneumonia *nil.*

9. That 105 uncomplicated cases, occurring consecutively in the clinical wards of the Royal Infirmary when under my care, during a period of 16 years, should all have recovered,

* These numerals correspond to those giving an abstract of the treatment in the previous pages of this section.

is a fact which can only be ascribed to the nature of the treatment, as is shown by contrasting the results of that treatment
with those of a lowering, expectant, mixed, or specific practice.

10. That just in proportion as other treatments approach
the restorative principle, and avoid lowering the system, so
much the greater is their success.   It will further be observed
that even where a direct lowering practice has been avoided,
if the diet has been restricted, or opium largely given, or
digitalis, alcohol, or other drug, tending to weaken the system
and diminish appetite employed, no great advantage has been
arrived at.   So that—

11. The variations which appear to follow the same treatment by different physicians are explicable by the amount of
weakness in the patient, or circumstances in the treatment
causing weakness, such as low diet, bleeding, tartar emetic,
narcotics, etc. etc.   It follows that supporting and restoring
(not stimulating) the nutritive powers of the system, and
avoiding all weakening remedies, ought to constitute the
practice in pneumonia.

PATHOLOGY OF ACUTE PNEUMONIA.

Pneumonia is a lesion consisting of liquor sanguinis poured
into the air vesicles, minute bronchial tubes, and parenchyma
of the lung.   The exudative process may be very limited,
indeed confined to a few air vesicles and the minute bronchial
tubes connected with them.   This is *vesicular pneumonia*. We
know it may be confined to a lobule or occupy an entire lobe,
constituting the so-called *lobular* and *lobar pneumonia*.   In
either case the essential phenomenon of inflammation—that is,
exudation—has occurred, distinguishable on careful examination of the pulmonary tissue, by the blocking up of air vesicles
with a finely-molecular matter.   Occasionally the vesicular

exudation may be felt on handling the lung in the form of
minute indurations, varying in size from a millet seed to that
of a pea—often red, but occasionally yellow, and in the latter
case very liable to be mistaken for tubercles. Such small
indurations, however, at length soften, and are converted into
pus, like the lobar and lobular forms of pneumonia.

Microscopic examination of the pulmonary tissue shows
us, in the first instance, that the air vesicles, the minute
bronchi, and the areolar tissue, are infiltrated with a molecular
and granular exudation, which often forms a complete cast or
mould of the vesicles and bronchi, easily separated mechani-
cally by washing and pressure. Not unfrequently, as was
shown by Remak, these moulds are expectorated entire, and
may be disengaged from the gelatinous matter with which
they are associated by throwing the contents of the spit-box
into water, and teazing out the branched filaments. These,
when magnified, present a fibrous exudation, in which are
imbedded commencing pus corpuscles, with a greater or less
number of epithelial cells. Such portions of exudation as
remain in the lung are transformed into pus, become ultimately
disintegrated and absorbed into the blood, where they are
chemically changed, and at length excreted from the system,
principally by the kidneys. If, from the extent of the disease or
weakness of the patient, this process is checked, the patient may
die, either from inability to excrete the effete matter which is
in the blood, or from interruption to the respiratory functions.
If the exudation be limited in extent, or have been poured
out slowly from the commencement, it may become what is
called chronic. Under such circumstances, the epithelial and
pus corpuscles of the pulmonary tissue may undergo the fatty
generation, and numerous compound granule cells be the result.
If blood should have been extravasated, mingled with the
other formations described, there will be often found red
crystals of hæmatine, blood corpuscles surrounded by an

albuminous layer, and presenting the numerous transformations which they are known to undergo after extravasation.

Dr. Todd* observes, "When a patient suffers from pneumonia, the tendency is for the lung to become solid, then for pus to be generated, and at last for the pus-infiltrated lung-structure to be broken down and dissolved. Such are the changes when matters take an unfavourable course. On the other hand, recovery takes place, either through the non-completion of the solidifying process or by the rapid removal, either through absorption or a process of solution and discharge of the new material, which had made the lung solid."

Now, I have directed special attention to the method in which the exudation is absorbed, and have frequently examined lungs after death in the stage of red hepatisation, where death had occurred from cerebral hæmorrhage or other disease. In some lungs there has been a pneumonia in all its stages, incipient in some places, solidified and red in others, grey and purulent in a third. In all these places a gradation in pus formation has been observable. In the most solid hepatisation young pus cells may be observed somewhere beginning to form ; so that I am convinced that the exudation is always broken down through the agency of purulent formation—in short, that this is the normal process. I have never seen any evidence that a coagulated exudation is simply disintegrated and absorbed without the development of pus cells, and I conceive that all analogy, as well as direct observation, is opposed to the supposition. It follows that, so far from the formation of pus being the evidence of an unfavourable course of the disease, it is the normal and necessary transformation of the solid exudation, whereby it is broken up and caused to be absorbed.

This view, based upon numerous careful histological examinations of pneumonic lungs, and easily capable of demon-

* Beale's Archives of Medicine. No. 1, p. 2.

stration in any recent specimen of the disease, as well as by
many preparations in my collection, shocks the notions of
certain pathologists of the French school. M. Grisolle recently
observes of it :—"I cannot accept a doctrine that is not justified by any direct proof, against which the clinical sense in a
manner revolts, and which is manifestly contrary to what has
been taught, and is still taught every day, by the simplest observation of physicians throughout the world."* If, before
writing such a criticism, M. Grisolle had investigated the
subject in the only way in which it can be investigated—
that is, with the microscope—he would have seen in red
hepatisation pus corpuscles in all stages of formation, and
thus convinced himself of a truth which, so far from revolting
the clinical sense, presents to it new and important arguments
for a more successful practice, as will be subsequently shown.
The microscope has proved that many so-called purulent
fluids are not purulent at all; whereas it distinctly demonstrates
that the disaggregation, softening, and liquefaction of the
plastic exudation in pneumonia—processes admitted by M.
Grisolle—are in truth the result of a vital growth of pus-cells ;
by favouring which we can cause recovery in our patients,
and by diminishing or interfering with which we increase the
mortality among them. The direct proof that M. Grisolle requires he may himself obtain by making a few sections of any
pneumonic lung with a Valentin's knife, and carefully examining them, first under a magnifying power of 25, and then of
250 diameters linear, when he will see appearances similar to
those now figured, and recognise—1st, Molecular exudation in
the air-vesicles ; 2d, Passage of this by molecular coalescence
into pus-cells ; and 3d, Formation and subsequent degener-
ation of such cells. Indeed, so constant is the production of
pus in pneumonia, and so clearly can it be seen to form by
molecular aggregation, independently of pre-existing cells, as

* Traité de la Pneumonie, 2me edit. 1864, p. 53.

in itself to carry with it a complete refutation of Virchow's doctrine, "omnis cellula e cellulâ," or what is commonly called "cell pathology."

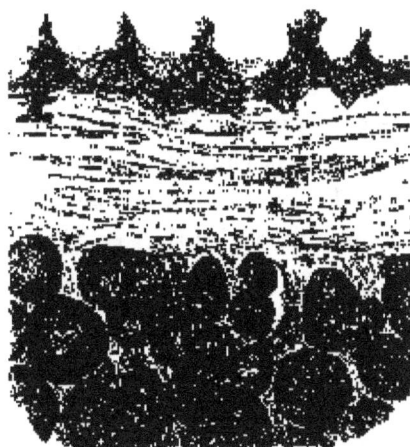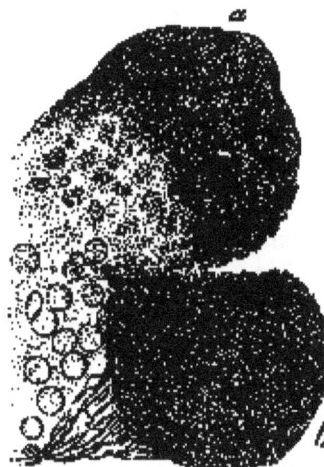

Fig. 1.   Fig. 2.

Fig. 1.—Vertical section through the outer portion of a lung affected with pleuro-pneumonia, magnified 25 diameters linear. Externally, the exudation on the surface has formed a thick layer of molecular fibres, and shows villi, which, on becoming vascular, absorb the serous fluid. The lower half of the figure shows the air vesicles of the lung blocked up with the coagulated molecular exudation.

Fig. 2.—Two air vesicles in red hepatisation of the lung, magnified 250 diameters linear. a, Filled with molecular exudation, aggregating into small masses to form pus corpuscles. b, A neighbouring air vesicle, in which the exudation has proceeded further in development, and is forming pus-cells.

The exudation having been transformed into pus-cells, these, after a time, become fatty, break down, disintegrate, and liquefy, and are absorbed into the blood, from whence they are excreted by the emunctories, but more especially by the kidneys, in the form of urates.

It is the pathology of the disease, as now explained, that many years ago forced upon my mind the conviction that blood-letting and antiphlogistics must be injurious. Pus-cells must be regarded as living growths, and as such require an excess of blood, good nutrition, and exalted vital force to hurry

on their development and carry them successfully through the
natural stages of their existence. If the resolution of a
pneumonia simply consisted of a retrograde process—of a so-
called necrosis of the exudation—an antiphlogistic practice, by
favouring it, might be expected to relieve the lung rapidly and
cure the disease. But my conviction, that such removal was
dependent upon vital processes of growth, led me to an
opposite treatment, viz., never to attempt cutting the disease
short, or to weaken the pulse and vital powers, but on the
contrary to further the necessary changes which the exudation
must undergo in order to be fully excreted from the economy.
To this end, during the period of febrile excitement I content
myself with giving salines in small doses with a view of
diminishing the viscosity of the blood. At the commencement
of the treatment I order as much beef-tea, milk, and other
nutrients as can be taken, and as soon as the pulse becomes
soft, solid food, and from 4 to 8 oz. of wine daily. As the
period of crisis approaches I give a diuretic, consisting of half
a drachm of nitric ether, and sometimes ten minims of colchi-
cum wine, three times daily, to favour excretion of urates.
But if crisis occurs by sweat or stool, I take care not to check
it in any way. I do not consider that the salines and diuretics
do more than assist the natural progress of the disease. The
essential part of the treatment consists in the rest, nourishment, and support given to the body throughout.

The object of this practice has been greatly misunderstood,
and by none more so than by M. Grisolle, who calls it an
expectant treatment. It seems to me to differ entirely from
it in the care which is taken to nourish the weakened frame
from the beginning, and thus, according to the pathological
views formerly explained, assist the vital powers to change
the coagulated exudation, first into a new growth (pus), and
then into a fluid capable of absorption. I cannot call it a
dietetic treatment, because this term has been applied on

the Continent to withholding diet rather than giving it—the "diete absolue" of the French, meaning starvation. This fact explains the fatal result of the practice, and especially the ill success of M. Grisolle, when he tried expectancy—or, as he understands by that method, withholding all nourishment—while at the same time the bowels are acted on by injections and castor-oil.* My pathology, in his opinion, appears strange, and useless to refer to ;† but as it has led me to cure every case of single and double uncomplicated pneumonia, whereas M. Grisolle's treatment produces a mortality of one in every six cases, I hope he will permit me to think that my theory is better founded on observation than he supposes, while my practice unquestionably supports its correctness.

I have dwelt very shortly on the pathology of Pneumonia in this place, because in the present state of science it can only be fully understood by entering at length into the great subject of inflammation. My object has been to point out that, so far as my own practice was concerned, I was led to it by scientific research. But now, after carefully observing and recording cases for seventeen years in the wards of an hospital, I venture to think that I am justified in maintaining that truth in practice coincides with truth in theory, and that the one supports and confirms the other.‡

OBJECTIONS ANSWERED.

In a question of great practical importance like the present, in which a procedure is recommended much opposed to past

* Traité de la Pneumonie, 2me edit. p. 559.
† Idem, p. 565.
‡ For a fuller consideration of the pathology of this subject the author would refer to the fourth edition of his Principles and Practice of Physic, 1855, more especially what is said under the heads of " Molecular and Cell Theories of Organisation " (p. 115); "Inflammation " (p. 155); "The natural Progress of Disease" (p. 295); and " On the Diminished Employment of Blood-letting and Antiphlogistic Remedies in the Treatment of Acute Inflammations " (p. 302).

experience, and to the opinions of many able physicians, it was not to be expected that no objections could be offered. Indeed these have been freely expressed, as the views now published have from time to time been made public in my lectures and writings. Without referring to these individually, I now propose to answer them under distinct heads.

OBJECTION 1. *No Plan of treating Pneumonia can be applicable to all Cases.*

A very general objection offered to the restorative plan of treatment in pneumonia is founded upon the presumed success of former modes of practice in cases peculiarly adapted to them. No one kind of treatment, it is said, can possibly be successful in all cases of pneumonia, inasmuch as some occur in robust and others in feeble constitutions. It has also been urged that the disease may occur under varied circumstances of age, sex, climate, constitution, etc., etc.; may present great differences in phenomena as regards pain, sleeplessness, breathlessness, expectoration, and so on; nay, more, the extent of the disease and its complications may give it peculiarities; and that all these will require variations in the treatment. These assertions appear not only fascinating, but most reasonable. It is even urged by many who have been obliged to admit the fatality of general blood-letting, tartar emetic, and antiphlogistics, that the cause of this is their not having been judiciously employed. If, it is argued, bleeding were only practised in such cases, and antimony, opium, and digitalis only given in such others, the result would have been different. Yet these and all such statements only constitute so many assumptions, wholly destitute of proof by those who make them.

Wherever, on the other hand, judicious medical men have practically acted on these ideas, although a marked improvement on the old antiphlogistic treatment has occurred, a considerable mortality has still taken place—which, when contrasted with the restorative treatment, exhibits the vast superiority of the latter. Thus we cannot doubt that these views have been ably carried out by Lebert, Huss, Bamberger, Flint, Rigler, and Morehead ; and yet a reference to p. 38 will prove that the highest success thus arrived at, which was by Lebert, is 1 death in 13 cases, and that, according to Huss, even uncomplicated cases so treated die in the proportion of 1 in 17 cases. To me, therefore, it appears certain that attempts to relieve particular symptoms by remedies which diminish strength and lessen appetite are objectionable, and that, although some patients may be apparently benefited, the practice as a rule should be avoided.

In reasoning with medical men who hold the objection here referred to, it will always be found that their arguments rest upon special cases. We have shown that where a strict antiphlogistic practice was the rule, one case of pneumonia in every three so treated died. This must be admitted to be a frightful mortality, occurring as it did in chosen uncomplicated cases, all of which, under a restorative treatment, may now be cured. But while one in three died, two in three recovered. If sixty cases had been treated, forty got well ; and the practitioner, in recounting the results of his practice in after years, dwells with complacency on the number of individuals he has saved with his lancet. These have made a strong impression on his mind. Those who died were forgotten. It must be clear that no correct conclusions can be arrived at as to the success of any treatment, unless all the cases are taken into consideration, and the number of fatal ones compared with those which recovered. When then it is assumed that vigorous or plethoric persons attacked with pneumonia require to be bled, whereas it is only the weak that should be supported,—where, I ask, is the proof of such

a dogma? In the same manner, when it is asserted that
excessive dyspnœa, or the disease attacking both lungs, de-
mands blood-letting,—where, I ask, is the proof? On the
other hand, I appeal to the facts tabulated at p. 12, *et seq.*, as
showing that both strong and weak individuals recover easily
under restoratives, and that the amount of dyspnœa, or the
disease attacking one or both lungs, in no way affects the
mortality.

That various circumstances greatly increase or diminish
the mortality and duration of pneumonia, has been proved
by various writers, but by no one more clearly than by Dr.
Sibson in his able article on this subject in the *Brit. and
For. Med. Chir. Review* for July 1858. The circumstances
he more especially alludes to are age, sex, and constitution of
the patient; the season, the climate, the previous destitution
of the patient, the early neglect of the disease, the extent,
character, and stage of the disease, the complications, the
change of type, and the hospital accommodation. Several of
his conclusions, looked at by the light of the facts I have now
published, require to be modified, especially those which refer
to the influence of the extent of the disease, and change of
type, which in truth produce little effect on the progress of
pneumonia. All the other circumstances may I think be
resolved under one head, viz., various causes producing weakness. Thus the reason that the disease is less fatal among young
persons under twenty than among adults or elderly people, is
evidently that they are more vigorous, and because the nutritive processes in them are more active. We have also seen
that among women, they being weaker than men, the disease is
more prolonged. In like manner, neglect of the disease at an
early period, and feebleness of constitution, as among the Hindoo
races, produce injurious effects. It should be noticed that the
observations of Dr. Sibson, and of other commentators, on a
past treatment, refer for the most part to the results of an outi-

phlogistic, expectant, or mixed treatment. We have shown that under a restorative treatment most of those circumstances which have been shown to affect pneumonia unfavourably are at once removed. The great fact that all my cases recovered except the four who died from fatal meningitis, ulcerated intestines, or kidney disease, shows that in this climate, under restoratives, age, sex, season, and constitution of the patient, have no influence on the mortality, although to some extent they affect the duration of the disease.

Perhaps there is no circumstance that influences the mortality and progress of a pneumonia more than neglect of the disease in its early stage. The lower classes not only starve themselves after the onset of the fever, but not unfrequently continue their work, until they become thoroughly exhausted, before entering an hospital. Such are the cases which when first seen are in a dying state, and which, if they do not die, have a prolonged convalescence. On the other hand, it is often remarkable how restoratives cause such individuals to rally and triumph over the disease. Thus, while in the strong, a restorative treatment enables them to pass quickly and safely through the malady, in the weak, it is the only method of averting death and securing recovery.

OBJECTION 2. *The Success of the Restorative Treatment is owing to a Change in the Type of the Disease.*

No sooner in 1848 had I commenced to make a trial of the restorative treatment of pneumonia in the clinical wards of the Royal Infirmary, than my very eminent colleague, the late Professor Alison, necessarily had it brought under his notice. Struck apparently with the results, so contrary to all his preconceived notions, he was led to the conclusion that they could only be explained by supposing that the type of inflammatory diseases had changed since the days of Cullen and Gregory. This

E

view he first put forth in his clinical lectures, delivered in
1850 and 1852, but more especially in a paper published in
1856,* and to which I replied at length in 1857.† This last
paper gave rise to what was called the blood-letting controversy of 1857 in this country, and which was even partici-
pated in on the continent and in the United States of America.
The theory put forth by Dr. Alison was, that the altered
practice in pneumonia and other acute diseases does not result from an improved knowledge or an advance in diagnosis
and pathology, but that these diseases themselves have changed.
He thought, for example, that inflammation is no longer the
same now that it was in the time of Cullen and Gregory ; that
the human constitution (in a manner which he did not explain)
is fundamentally altered, and has become weaker; so that
medical men were as right in treating disease by blood-letting
in former days as they are now in abstaining from it. So
satisfactory did this theory appear to its founder, that he
claimed for it the dignity of an ultimate fact or axiom. Thus,
says Dr. Alison, changes of type in inflammatory diseases
constitute a "part of the general dispensations of Providence
as to those diseases, and are, as far as yet known, an *ultimate
fact in their history.*" Dr. Watson says, no less emphatically,
in the last edition of his work on the "Practice of Physic :"
"I am firmly persuaded, by my own observations, and by the
records of medicine, that there are waves of time through
which the sthenic and the asthenic characters of disease prevail in succession ; and that we are at present living amid one
of its adynamic phases."

* "Reflections on the results of experience as to the symptoms of internal
inflammations, and the effects of blood-letting, during the last forty years"
(*Edin. Med. Journal*).
† "Observations on the results of an advanced diagnosis and pathology,
applied to the management of internal inflammations, compared with the
effects of a former antiphlogistic treatment, and especially of blood-letting."
—(*Edin. Med. Journal*, vol. ii. p. 769.)

Let us for a moment consider what this theory implies—viz., that the constitution of mankind has become weaker and less capable of bearing depletion now than formerly; that the human pulse, by which this is tested, beats less vigorously when diseased than it did for hundreds of years before the days of Cullen and Gregory; that when a strong man, now-a-days, is seized with an inflammation, he presents all the phenomena that used to be observed in a weak one: in short, that the human race has so degenerated during the last five-and-thirty years that the reaction which formerly used to take place in the economy no longer occurs, and that it cannot bear depletion so well.

But surely this idea may be said to repose on no facts whatever, but merely on supposition; for, when we investigate the effects of injuries after the battle of Waterloo and after the battle of the Alma, we find them, in the British army, identically the same. Neither has any change been observed in this respect in our civil hospitals. Further, the people, generally, are better fed, clothed, and housed than they used to be; the comforts and enjoyments of life are far more widely diffused, and its absolute value, according to the bills of mortality, is greatly augmented. Our mental strength, commercial enterprise, engineering skill, martial daring, and bodily vigour might easily be shown never to have surpassed what this country can now boast of—facts entirely opposed to this theory.

The treatment of inflammation without antiphlogistics has also been introduced among veterinary practitioners. Is it to be maintained, therefore, that our horses and cattle have, as the result of civilisation, been enervated, and that in them, also, the type of disease is altered? We nowhere observe this any more among them than among mankind; they still draw the same loads—still plough with the same depth of furrow—still run with the same if not greater speed.

Besides, it should not be forgotten that the antiphlogistic was a fatal practice—in acute pneumonia amounting to one death in from three to six cases (I.-IV.) In my wards there were no deaths in similar uncomplicated cases under a restorative treatment. To prove that this is a result of treatment, and not of change of type, it is only necessary to consider that, in countries such as Spain and Italy, where the old practice is still followed, it produces the same fatal result. Have we not all recently been startled by the death of Count Cavour, which followed five bleedings for a fever? It surely will not be maintained that whilst the people of Britain, France, and Germany have degenerated, those of Spain and Italy have retained their pristine vigour? In Paris M. Bouillaud continues to pursue his system of bleeding by the *coup-sur-coup* method. He is the only one in that capital who does so. Can we, on this account, believe that in his wards the type of disease has not changed, whilst in every other hospital and ward it has? On the contrary, we find that wherever large bleedings are practised at present, the same great mortality exists which formerly prevailed—showing that the disease is unaltered.

Then it has been argued that epidemic fevers change their type, and so they unquestionably do, but it in no way follows that organic diseases should do so likewise. The morbid poisons in the atmosphere, arising from various sources, are more powerful at one period than another, and not only induce symptoms varying in intensity, but cause varied symptoms, such as occur in typhus and typhoid fevers. It is the latter changes which constitute difference in type. But there have been strong and weak men in all ages ; while blows, injuries, and changes of temperature have similarly affected them, occasioning symptoms proportioned to their bodily vigour, but in no way altering the character of the symptoms themselves. Have cancer, tubercle, or other structural changes undergone a change of type? Tubercular diseases of the lung were until lately considered to be almost always fatal; now, owing to an improved treatment, it is known that they frequently recover. Are we therefore to believe that, while persons affected with inflammations are weaker, those affected with phthisis and scrofula are stronger than they used to be?

But it is stated that the pulse has altered: formerly it was found to be strong, now it is comparatively weak. Why, within the last twenty-five years nature should have changed the pulse of man and animals is not very clear. Judging from the circumstances to which I have alluded, especially the more abundant food and prosperity of the people, it ought to be stronger instead of weaker. But some have already brought forward ideas to explain the supposititious fact. Thus it has been said the use of tea instead of malt-liquor, spirits, and wine, renders people weaker and more nervous. Some have thought that the use of potatoes, and others the employment of railways, has something to do with it. Dr. Watson is of opinion that it is attributable to the epidemics of cholera, which, in a manner he has not sought to explain, "leave traces of their operation on the health and vitality of a community long after they have ceased to prevail as epidemics." (*Pneumonia*, vol. ii p. 97.) Mr. Robertson of Manchester is satisfied from experience that it is the boil epidemic which has caused this remarkable change of type. Some suppose that it is dependent on the altered relations between our urban and rural populations. Would it not be well for those who are already discussing the causes of a change that is by no means apparent, to ask themselves, in the first instance, how they establish the fact that the pulse is changed at all?

I need scarcely say that memory and mere opinion in a case of this kind are not of much value. How often do our senses deceive us when objects are at hand; how little can

they be depended on when it is simply asserted that in the
memory of this or that practitioner a pulse was stronger
twenty years ago than it is now. And yet we have no
further evidence than this advanced by the supporters of a
theory which claims as its fundamental fact a diminished
vital force in the heart and pulse of man and animals, to
explain a change of practice. But what say science and positive
observation to these assertions? It so happens that there is no
subject in all physiology with regard to which we possess more
elaborate and more exact information than we do concerning
the pulse. In 1732 Stephen Hales published a remarkable
series of experiments regarding the static force of the pulse,
and the rapidity of the blood through arteries of different
calibres. In 1828-29 similar observations were made by
Poisseulle with an instrument invented for that purpose,
which he called the "hæmadynamometer," that led him to the
same conclusion as that arrived at by Hales. In these
experiments the force of the pulse was determined by the
height to which the impulse of the blood could elevate a column
of mercury. It resulted that the static force with which the
blood is impelled in the human aorta is equal to the pressure
of 4 lb. 4 oz. on the square inch, and in the radial pulse is
equal to about 4 drachms. Valentine confirmed these results
in 1844, Ludwig in 1847, and Vierordt so late as 1855; so
that not only is there no fact whatever in support of the
notion that the pulse of man or animals is weaker now than
formerly, but all positive researches during a period of one
hundred and thirty years prove the very contrary. It appears
to me, therefore, that the theory of change of type, so far from
being established on well-known facts, is, on the contrary,
altogether erroneous, being entirely opposed to the accurate
data which histology, physiology, and pathology have accumu-
lated in modern times.

I would refer the readers interested in this subject to a

detailed analysis of the papers which appeared during the blood-letting controversy of 1857, in the third edition of my "Principles and Practice of Medicine," 1859, p. 297. The preceding summary of the argument is reprinted from the fourth edition, 1865. While these pages, however, are passing through the press, Professor Stokes of Dublin has added his distinguished name to those of the physicians who have contended strongly for a change of type in pneumonia during the last thirty or forty years. He says : " I well remember observing the frequent occurrence of the phenomena mentioned by Dr. Christison—the vehement action of the heart, the incompressibility of the pulse, the vivid redness of the venous blood, and the force with which it spouted, almost *per saltum* from the orifice in the vein."* It must be regarded as a singular circumstance, that whilst Dr. Stokes is appealing to his memory in order to support the theory of change of type, Dr. G. Balfour should publish a paper in which he quotes the cases of Cullen and Gregory, from notes of their Lectures preserved in the libraries of the Edinburgh College of Physicians and of the London Medico-Chirurgical Society. These records of cases taken at the time, distinctly prove that the pneumonia which occurred in their day presented exactly the same type as pneumonia does now. In most of the cases the pulse was soft. Indeed, so far from the pulse being strong and incompressible, as it was according to the memories of Drs. Christison and Stokes, Dr. Gregory lays it down as a rule that " in respect to the fulness of the pulse in pneumonia in the beginning before the patient was blooded, it is not only soft but small ; but commonly after the patient is blooded it becomes fuller, although it always retains its softness."†
Surely positive facts written down at the bed-side during the life of the patient must constitute more valuable evidence of

* Address in Medicine to the British Medical Association, 1865.
† Edinburgh Medical Journal, September 1865, p. 216.

what really existed, than mere remembrances of the past by physicians, however eminent. It follows that the change of practice in modern times cannot be ascribed to change of pulse and a typhoid type of disease, as has been supposed.

Another statement of Dr. Stokes will, I venture to think, on inquiry be found in no way to support his doctrine. Alluding to the appearances presented by pneumonia in specimens presented to the Pathological Society of Dublin in recent times, as compared with the years 1820-30, he says: "As a general rule these specimens all showed appearances indicative of a less degree of pathologic energy. In pneumonia, for example, the redness, firmness, compactness, and defined boundary of the solidified lung was seldom seen; and that state of dryness and vivid scarlet injection to which I venture to give the name of the first stage of pneumonia became very rare. In place of these characters, we had a condition more approaching to splenisation, the affected parts purple, not bright red; friable, not firm; moist, not dry; and the whole looking more like the result of diffuse than of energetic and concentrated inflammation; or we had another form, to which Dr. Corrigan has given the name of blue pneumonia, in which the structure resembled that of a carnified lung, which had been steeped in venous blood." Accepting the facts as detailed by Dr. Stokes, they admit of easy explanation without the necessity of supposing that organic alterations of the human frame have in recent times undergone any sensible alteration in their physical characters. In the first place, in consequence of an improved treatment very few persons now die in the first stage of pneumonia, a circumstance quite sufficient to account for the rarity of that solid and defined red hepatisation of the lung to which Dr. Stokes has alluded. But every pathologist must be aware that when he does examine a primary uncomplicated pneumonia in the early stage, it presents exactly the same aspect and characteristics now as it always did. In the second place,

there can be no doubt that the greater frequency with which
post-mortem examinations are now performed, and the increased attention which has been paid to morbid anatomy,
have brought to light lesions which were formerly little understood, such as splenisations, carnifications, and collapses of the
lung. It must be evident, however, that the decrease in
number of true examples of firm red hepatisation, and the
apparent increase of the splenisations and softer lesions of the
organs so frequent in fevers, is no proof of change in the same
lesion, but rather of a lessened mortality of the one disease, and
a consequent comparative increase of the others.

Dr. Stokes further denies that an advanced diagnosis and
pathology have had any influence in reducing the mortality in
cases of acute pneumonia. As to diagnosis, he asserts that no
improvement has taken place since the days of Laennec. But
while this may be admitted in the sense that Laennec and
a few of his followers could detect pneumonia physically
as well as physicians can now, it must also be conceded that
the skill they possessed is at present far more widely diffused
among medical men, and that practically such extension of
diagnostic power has greatly contributed to give precision
in detecting the disease. As to the influence of cell pathology,
I have from the first maintained that it was the consideration
that pus cells were vital formations, through the agency of
which the exudation was removed, that led me to change my
own practice. This pathology, however, as previously explained (see p. 47, *et seq.*), has nothing to do with the cell
pathology of Virchow, with which it has been strangely
mingled by Dr. Stokes. The doctrine of Virchow is that
every cell springs from a pre-existing cell, and arises in no
other way, and that we must not transfer the seat of real
action to any point beyond the cell. To this doctrine I have
always been opposed, and shown that there exist such striking facts proving the existence of vital action without cells at
all, as to render the hypothesis of Virchow untenable—the

pus cells, for example, which infiltrate the lung in cases of pneumonia may readily be shown to originate independent of previously existing cells. On these important points, however, I cannot here enter at further length, but would refer the reader to a series of lectures I published in the *Lancet* on molecular physiology, pathology, and therapeutics, during 1863, and to a short account of molecular and cell theories of organisation, p. 115 of the last edition of my "Principles and Practice of Medicine." It must, I think, be clear that it is to the law of nutrition, as arrived at by the cultivation of histology, that we are indebted for the present theory of inflammation, and for the successful practice which has been founded upon it.

In the whole of this discussion I have endeavoured to avoid saying anything that could wound the feelings of those who formerly employed antiphlogistics in the treatment of pneumonia. My object has not been to show—as my esteemed friend Dr. Stokes seems to think—that our "predecessors were deficient in observation and erroneous in practice." On the contrary, I believe that former physicians were thoroughly conscientious, and acted in perfect harmony with the pathology of their day, and the then state of knowledge. But now that pathology has greatly advanced, and our knowledge has been correspondingly extended, it surely becomes us, instead of remaining slaves to the authority of our forefathers, to imitate them at least in this—viz., to bring our theory and practice into harmony with one another. My real purpose has been to demonstrate that our acquaintance with diseased processes has led us to a treatment which has greatly diminished the mortality of acute inflammations, and if I have succeeded I shall rejoice that the end has been obtained, while I regret that such eminent physicians as Drs. Alison, Christison, Watson, and Stokes have differed with me in opinion.

OBJECTION 3. *Bleeding should still be employed under certain circumstances.*

In my paper in 1857, when demonstrating the injurious effects of bleeding and antiphlogistics on the mortality and duration of pneumonia, I took great pains to point out that these remedies unquestionably relieved symptoms, and might, therefore, in appropriate circumstances, if used cautiously, be employed as palliatives. I said, "But whilst large and repeated bleedings, practised with a view of arresting the disease, appear to me opposed to a correct pathology, small and moderate bleedings, directed to palliate certain symptoms, and especially excessive pain and dyspnœa, may reasonably be had recourse to, and, unless there be great weakness, without any fear of doing injury. I have often been struck, especially in cases where large thoracic aneurisms cause these symptoms, with the small loss of blood which will occasion marked relief. The same result may be hoped for in other cases where the congestion is passive, even when this is associated with active repletion of blood, followed by exudation. But I need scarcely remark that this mere palliative object of blood-letting is not the ground on which the practice has hitherto been based, and that in this point of view it requires to be very differently explained."

And again, "There are cases, which were formerly often mistaken for inflammation, in which blood-letting may still be useful. I allude to those where an obstruction to the circulation exists in the heart and lung dependent on over-distension of the right side of the former organ, and cases of venous congestion, engorgement, and perhaps œdema of the latter; also certain cases of bronchitis preventing aeration, of aneurisms, and of asphyxia. Although even here the true value of the remedy has yet to be positively ascer-

tained, the special cases demanding it more carefully dis-
criminated, and the mechanical principles which justify the
practice determined. The temporary benefit occasioned in
many of these cases by the loss of a trifling amount of blood
is often very remarkable, and has been previously referred to.
I have seen instances where great dyspnœa and pain, caused
by large thoracic aneurisms in vigorous men, have been greatly
alleviated, and inexpressible relief produced for from twelve
to twenty-four hours, by a bleeding to the extent of only five
ounces. It seems probable that this may arise from diminishing for a time the tension of the whole vascular system.
But whatever be the explanation of this fact, I hold that, as
a palliative, and practised to a limited extent in cases where
no great debility exists, blood-letting may still be had recourse
to. So with regard to antimonials, although in the large
doses, which weaken the heart and force of the pulse, they
are not serviceable, in smaller doses, together with other
neutral salts, they may assist in diminishing the viscosity of
the blood, and in favouring the excretion of the effete matters
by the skin and kidneys."

To these views I still adhere, although of late years I
have never found it necessary to have recourse to blood-letting even as a palliative, having found that warm poultices
locally produce just as much relief.

Another passage from my original paper in 1857 deserves
consideration here :—" It has been argued that the immediate
beneficial effects of blood-letting justify the practice. This is a
therapeutical question of the greatest importance, and one which
I venture to think has not been sufficiently considered by
medical men. No doubt pain is a great evil, and mankind
instinctively seek for relief, and sometimes at any cost.
But if the possession of life be an advantage, it is ofttimes
only to be maintained at the price of suffering more or less
privation and pain. It is in this point of view that disease

may frequently be considered as a benefit and a great good, mercifully sent by a wise Providence to reconcile man under a variety of circumstances to death itself, as to a great relief. But such is not the therapeutical or curative method of considering the question ; the great object of the physician being *first* to cure, and, should his attempts in that direction fail, *then* to relieve. If both objects can be accomplished, so much the better ; but if the means of relief are opposed to those of cure, then to obtain the latter the former must be unhesitatingly sacrificed. I have pointed out in another place how much this principle has been overlooked in the treatment of pulmonary consumption ;[*] and in no case does it appear to have been more disregarded than in inflammation. For assuming it as granted that in some cases the pain is for a time relieved by bleeding, and that in pneumonia the respiration temporarily becomes more free, at what a cost are these advantages obtained should the patient be so weakened as to be unable to rally. Even if he does rally, a large bleeding almost always prolongs the disease. I do not consider it necessary to cite cases in proof of the fact, that in many instances bleeding has done great mischief, because this will be readily admitted by all candid medical men."

Very recently it has been contended by Dr. Markham, that under those circumstances which, from the first, I pointed out, admitted of very limited bleedings of four or five ounces, venesection until the patient shows *signs of relief or of fainting* is not merely a palliative, but, to use his own language, "a most sovereign and life-saving remedy." Now, to carry bleeding so far as this, is in my opinion injurious and unnecessary, from four to eight ounces being quite sufficient. In a healthy man at 36, with double pleuro-pneumonia, accompanied by pain and dyspnœa (nothing said of the pulse), Dr. Markham

[*] The Pathology and Treatment of Pulmonary Consumption, by the Author. Edinburgh 1859, 2d edit., p. 143, *et seq.*

took sixteen ounces of blood from the patient by venesection, to his very great and immediate relief, a week after the onset of the disease. The pain in the right side returned again in the evening, and therefore eight or ten leeches were then applied. Next morning the man was comparatively in a most comfortable state. "But," it is observed, "I do not intend to follow out the history of this man's case through his long convalescence. I will only add, that in addition to the double pneumonia, he was afterwards attacked with pericarditis; and that subsequently a pleuritic abscess of the right side opened into and discharged its contents through the lungs and the trachea." Instead of having doubts, however, as to the value of the remedy in this case, it is confidently stated that "the man would have perished had he not been bled."

The clinical lecture of Dr. Markham on this and another case concludes as follows:—"Let no theoretical arguing draw us away from the patent fact which we have seen with our eyes. We saw a man, to all appearance *in extremis*, fighting an unequal battle with disease. We found him to be a subject of pleuro-pneumonia. We saw an immediate stop, then and there, put to the violence of this deadly struggle by bleeding. We saw the man recover from the moment of the bleeding. You may have heard him declare that the bleeding was the saving of his life, though you need not, perhaps, take any great account of a patient's opinion on such a point. You have seen all this. I think a man must be sceptical indeed, beyond all bounds of reason and common-sense (if I may invoke that sense here), who refuses to connect effect with causation, the consequence with the antecedent, the cure of the disease with the venesection, in the cases which I have brought under your notice. And this one other word let me add suggestively, what other remedy do you know of under the sun which is capable of producing off-hand, then and there, such great results in such formidable disease?"*

This eulogistic praise of blood-letting is exactly the same in kind as was employed thirty years ago, and results from a similar observation of the immediate relief produced by the remedy, irrespective of its dangers and subsequent effects. Although the healthy man of 36 had a lingering convalescence, although pericarditis and pleuritic abscess followed, these were esteemed to be of little moment. The pneumonia is assumed to be a formidable disease, the dyspnœa, so common in double cases from the fourth to the seventh day, is described as placing the man *in extremis*, and the "unequal battle with disease," "the deadly struggle," is at once put a stop to by bleeding ! Now, in my opinion the real danger which this patient was exposed to arose from the pericarditis, pleuritic abscess, and subsequent exhaustion. Why should a man in health be attacked by such sequelæ ? Were they caused by the bleeding and leeches employed on the seventh day, when he was already prostrated by a week's fever ? Might not the loss of four or five ounces of blood have produced all the palliative effects of the larger quantity taken ? Might not a warm poultice locally, with an etheroal draught and nourishment, have put him into as comfortable a state next morning without bleeding at all ? How can it be shown that this man, with his lingering convalescence, and his subsequent pericarditis and pleuritic abscess, was in any way benefited by bleeding ? Might it not be argued more consistently with the dictates of "reason and common-sense," that a proper connection of "effect with causation" would demonstrate that the patient gained a temporary palliation at a risk which nearly cost him his life ?

To answer these questions correctly, let us leave assumptions and glowing descriptions, and attend to the sober facts exhibited in our tabulated cases. Among these were thirty cases of double pneumonia, all of whom recovered, and the effects of bleeding upon them will be observed by running the eye over those distinguished by the letter D in the second column. It is a most instructive fact, that wherever bleeding was practised in those cases prostration supervened, and the convalescence was greatly prolonged; whereas, in every case where the patient was healthy, as in the man treated by Dr. Markham, notwithstanding the most urgent dyspnœa and pain, recovery under restoratives was rapid and perfect (see Cases VI., XLIV., and LXXI., and contrast them with Cases X., XIV., XXXVIII., L., LI., LIV., LVII., LXX., LXXV., CXIII.)

As a contrast to the case of Dr. Markham, Case XXXVIII. may be referred to (see Table, p. 14). A robust man, æt. 51, in whom both lungs were affected, with lividity of face and intense dyspnœa. He also might have been described to be "*in extremis*, fighting an unequal battle with disease." He was not bled; had nutrients and stimulants; and instead of a lingering convalescence, with pericarditis and pleuritic abscess, was quite well and left the hospital in nine days (see also Appendix, Cases V. to VIII.)

A still more important lesson, however, may be derived from this discussion—viz. that in medicine no sound conclusion can be drawn from the glowing description of a few cases in illustration of any treatment whatever. Sober facts, well attested and tabulated, are what we require, with all the leading phenomena of the disease accurately observed and recorded. More especially, it is necessary for arriving at truth to give a series of cases in which the failures as well as the successes are considered, avoiding all assumptions and rhetorical efforts, and depending alone upon completeness and exactitude of detail.

In a subsequent paper on this subject * Dr. Markham explains that he would only bleed in those cases of pneumonia in which the respiration is seriously interfered with. He further seeks to draw a distinction between bleeding with, and bleeding without, starvation, and certainly, as either pro-

* Brit. Med. Journal, vol. i. 1865, p. 477.

cooling is bad, both together are doubly so. The latter, however, he seems to think, so far from being bad, is, as we have seen, "a most sovereign and life-saving remedy." This I cannot admit, for in the face of the facts I have referred to it cannot be shown that it saves life. It *does* temporarily relieve pain and dyspnœa, but if it prolong the convalescence, and give rise to such sequelæ as pericarditis and pleuritic abscess, can it be said to be free from danger?

Dr. Markham further remarks—" When Professor Bennett talks of the dangers attending the loss of a few ounces of blood in pneumonia, I cannot help asking him to explain how it is that we daily see so many patients in hospital, surgical and medical, the feeble as well as the strong, losing without apparent injury, and often—and especially in lung and heart diseases—to their very great relief, large quantities of blood? What proof do these very numerous facts daily under our eyes afford of the danger of the loss of a few ounces of blood?"

This kind of argument and of questioning have been made to support the worst practice that could be devised. I have already pointed out that when 1 person in every 3 died of pneumonia, the large number that recovered was constantly appealed to in support of the antiphlogistic practice (p. 55). The idea, therefore, that bleedings, to the extent implied by Dr. Markham (that is, "until the patient shows signs of relief or of fainting"), may be practised with impunity, not to talk of benefit, is disproved by all known facts, and cannot be overthrown by vague statements as to the large number who recover (See Appendix, Case VIII.) The question should be—not how many recover, but how many die? and if Dr. Markham will show that in his hospital 100 cases of pneumonia with dyspnœa have been bled—as he advises—consecutively without a single death, he will do much to solve the practical question at issue. Even then, to establish that it is superior to a

F

plan of restoratives without bleeding, it would be necessary
to prove that the amount of re'ief obtained more than coun-
terbalanced the weakness which renders residence in a hospital much longer.

The whole of this discussion strongly indicates how necessary it is that we should emancipate ourselves from confident
plausibilities and fallacious assumptions. When a highly
respected and experienced medical man asserts that he has
found this or that practice advantageous, what does he mean?
He should point out in what way or to what extent it is advantageous, and how it influences the mortality and duration
of disease. Yet how seldom is this attempted to be done.
No stronger authority, no more illustrious names in medicine,
can be found than what supported the practice of venesection
and antiphlogistics in pneumonia. Yet the most rigorous
proof has shown us that they were utterly unconscious of the
great mortality among the cases they treated, and regarded a
recovery of 2 cases out of 3 as a triumph of their art. It
follows, that to determine results we must count our cases,
number the bad with the good ones, and instead of viewing
medical practice from the one-sided aspect of what is apparently successful, sternly determine to give the unfavourable
results a prominent place in the picture. This leads me to
consider—

OBJECTION IV. *Statistics are incapable of determining the
value of treatment.*

On no subject does the contradictory character of medical
reasoning become more apparent than on that of medical
statistics; because, whilst every practitioner is constantly
endeavouring to multiply those cases which seem to prove
his treatment to be successful, he regards with aversion every-
thing that reminds him of failure. Nothing is more common

than to see all sorts of remedies recommended to our notice on the faith of a few apparently good cases, whereas nothing is so rare as to find careful records of treatment in a series of cases, including the failures. How common, also, is the tendency to ascribe recoveries to medical skill, while the deaths are referred to the inevitable progress of the malady. Although philosophical physicians have in all times pointed out the fallacy of these beliefs, they still hold almost universal sway over the medical profession. The descriptions of systematic writers on medicine have tended to foster this state of things, in which we find accounts of maladies neatly divided into stages, forms, and varieties, and a treatment recommended—said to be successful according to experience—much of which, however, when tested clinically, is soon recognised to be inconsistent with reality. There is only one method of extrication from the difficulties so created, and that is by numbering and analysing well-recorded cases. In every proposition regarding the treatment of disease, we cannot avoid the consideration involved in statistics. It is no argument to say that they may be defective. If so, they must be rendered exact; and cases must be carefully taken, rigorously collected, and critically analysed. In no other way can we guard ourselves against representations of sanguine persons, generalisations from imperfect data, and confident assertions and assumptions based on the memory of success and the forgetfulness of failure.

The great objection always brought against medical statistics is the limited number of the facts from which conclusions are drawn. No one observer, it is argued, is capable of collecting a sufficient number of cases to enable him to derive exact information from them. Dr. Barclay, in a work entitled "Medical Errors," has recently endeavoured to support this view by an algebraical formula, which leads him to the conclusion that, if variable circum-

stances exist to the number of 15 in any given disease, no
less than 32,000 cases would be required before we could
meet with two of them exactly alike. He goes on to point
out that these variable circumstances, such as differences in
time, place, age, etc., oppose an insurmountable obstacle to
obtaining similarity in cases. But it may be asked, is such
exactitude in every particular necessary? because, if so, it
might just as reasonably be argued that we ought not only
to avoid comparing cases which occur in different countries and
cities, but also in different houses, or even beds. The line of
argument adopted by Dr. Barclay might apply to the chances
of meeting with exactly the same combination of numbers in
throwing ten or fifteen dice, but is wholly inapplicable and
out of place in reference to medical cases. It is well observed by Louis* that the leaf of a tree having been well described, can always be recognised. It is not necessary, in
order to compare one tree with another, that every individual
leaf on each be identical in size and form. So with diseases :
the essential characters admit of being known and so compared with one another as to allow the formation of general
laws, which every-day experience confirms.

But Dr. Barclay declares that an attempt lately made to
obtain a large number of cases of pneumonia by the aid of
the British Medical Association can lead to little benefit;
because, among other reasons, "acute pneumonia is just one
of those diseases in which a certain number of individuals
attacked will die, in spite of any treatment yet known, while
a certain number will recover if entirely left to themselves."
The assumptions contained in this one sentence afford an excellent example of loose reasoning, and of the necessity of
that statistical knowledge which the author condemns. What
entitles Dr. Barclay to affirm that a certain number of indi-

* See his admirable memoir on the numerical method, in the first volume
of the *Mémoires de la Société Médicale d'Observation*, p. 28.

viduals attacked will die in spite of any treatment yet known? The statement is evidently a gratuitous assumption, and begs the very question at issue. Its correctness is opposed by the fact, demonstrated in these pages, that 105 consecutive cases of primary and uncomplicated pneumonia under a restorative treatment all recovered. Should he not, consistently with his own argument, instead of opposing the employment of statistics among the members of the British Medical Association, urge them to second my endeavours? For if, according to his calculations, 32,000 cases be required, and the members of that Association number 2500, only 13 cases from each, instead of the 129 I have myself furnished, would serve to solve the problem in his own way. I believe, however, that 100 well-recorded consecutive cases, and in some instances half that number, are amply sufficient to test the value of any therapeutical remedy whatever.

Dr. Barclay, after pointing out the necessity of extreme similarity in the cases which are to be compared, and fully admitting the propriety of not "jumbling together the different experiences and cases of different practitioners," refers to the able paper of Dr. Sibson formerly alluded to, who has collected statistics of pneumonia from various sources, and given them in a tabular form, divided into two columns, headed, "Bleeding and Non-Bleeding Plan" respectively. Of this he remarks : " Although he (Dr. S.) draws various conclusions from a strict analysis of all that admit of it, he does not even sum up the figures which he gives as a whole." But what Dr. Sibson as a good statistician did not do, knowing well the absurdity of adding together cases which, although bled or not bled, differed widely otherwise with regard to their treatment, Dr. Barclay actually does, with the following result : "Of 1750 patients, treated by repeated or large bleedings, the mortality was 18.5 per cent. Of about 1000 treated by few and small bleedings, it was 13.5 per cent.

Taking both these together, the cases in which blood-letting formed one part of the treatment gave a death rate of 164 in the thousand; while 10,000 cases, treated almost entirely without venesection, gave a death rate of 203 in the thousand." It is thus made to appear that bleeding in pneumonia causes only 164 deaths, while non-bleeding increases the mortality to 203 deaths in the thousand. So that Dr. Barclay, with a view of showing the fallacy of medical statistics, violates the rules he himself admits to be necessary, and then points to the absurd conclusion in vindication of his argument.

This mode of reasoning, though very common, is entirely fallacious, and has led the author of "Medical Errors" to one of the most erroneous conclusions ever arrived at in modern times. This will be at once admitted on observing, that among the cases he adds together as treated by the non-bleeding plan, the treatment otherwise was quite different. Some of them were treated by antimonials in large doses, others by calomel, others by opium, others by digitalis, others by chloroform, others by metallic tonics, others by starvation, and others by restoratives. Above all, in his list of cases not bled more than one-half are derived from the general returns of hospitals, including many that entered moribund, so that the mortality amongst this class is very large. It is by adding such incongruous materials together the result is made to appear that there are fewer deaths amongst such as were bled than amongst those that were not. Such a statistic applied to determine the value of bleeding or non-bleeding in pneumonia can only mislead, for no correct conclusion can be derived from a series of cases in which, while some are and others are not bled, the mortality is influenced by other powerful drugs and modes of treatment. Instead, therefore, of showing the fallacy of medical statistics by this example, all that Dr. Barclay proves is the error which results from their wrong application.

Dr. Barclay objects to my statistics "that it is impossible to find any one circumstance *invariably* present or absent in the series of recoveries or deaths which in the least degree accounts for the termination one way or the other."[*] But he previously says—"Probably all had nutrients, by which I suppose beef-tea, milk, etc.—in fact, *food* is meant. But the fact is stated with reference to some, and not to others." Dr. Barclay has evidently not observed a passage referring to the table, p. 22, in which I state what is meant by nutrients, and that, though not specially mentioned, they were given in all cases. Here, then, is the invariable fact he required, which accounts in my opinion for the large number of recoveries, as fully explained in answer to Objection 1, p. 54. To this I consider the success to be owing, such various remedies as were employed being either innocuous or palliative, or, as in the case where depressants and starvation were used, by diminishing strength, tending to delay recovery. The deaths, as we have seen, were not caused by the pneumonia, but by fatal complications in other organs.

Both Dr. Barclay and Dr. Markham also object to certain reservations I have made in my statistics. "Why," says the former, "should a case partly treated by a colleague be withheld, when a case bled, blistered, and purged before admission is included?" To this I reply, that I could not conscientiously include in my series examples of pneumonia in which the treatment I advocate was not tried or was frustrated. For example : On taking charge of the clinical wards I find a man sinking who had been treated antiphlogistically and largely bled under a colleague. He shortly afterwards dies under my care, and I witness the post-mortem examination, which the pathologist records as a case of simple pneumonia, fatal in my hands. Surely Dr. Barclay will not maintain that to be a fair illustration of the effects of my practice.

* Brit. Med. Journal, Nov. 11, 1865.

Again: A case is admitted under my care which proceeds satisfactorily, but on giving up the wards to a colleague it is treated by calomel and opium, and a prolonged convalescence occurs. For this I am in no degree responsible, and cannot consider the case as one treated by me. But when persons who have been reduced by bleeding, purging, or mercurials, enter my wards, and rally and recover under restoratives, then I consider such case as one which legitimately belongs to my series. It is true some may argue that the cause of recovery is to be sought in the previous lowering treatment—an opinion that can only be confirmed or nullified by studying other cases, and by multiplying observations.

What is really required is that cases should be carefully observed and recorded by hospital physicians on a uniform plan. I still venture to think that, with reference to treatment, the facts recorded in the schedule issued to the members of the British Association are amply sufficient, and that they are easily arrived at. They are exactly the same as those in which I have recorded my own cases (see p. 12, *et seq.*) If others would follow the same plan, it is clear comparisons might be instituted, and all the essential sources of error avoided.

I cannot help thinking that the slight trouble required, and the general want of interest which prevails on such topics amongst the members of an overtaxed profession, are the real causes which led to the failure of the attempt in 1863.[*] A few also were doubtful as to whether cases of pure pneumonia, uncomplicated with pleurisy, bronchitis, or other disease, were required. It seldom happens that a pneumonia exists independent of some bronchitic or pleuritic affection; but this, if slight, in no way affects the result. If, on the other hand, it be intense, so that the pneumonia be secondary

---

[*] I may observe that only 15 members of the British Medical Association returned their schedules to me, containing 45 cases of Pneumonia.

in importance, this, if recorded, must be stated in the appropriate column, and all error will be avoided in collecting the cases.

I still hope that the sanction of large numbers may be given to the views contained in these pages, so that a great practical subject in medicine may be finally settled. We might then hope that a similar investigation might afford trustworthy results in other diseases; and thus the practice of our art approximate more towards uniformity. It must be admitted that mere assertion and opinion are altogether incapable of determining any question whatever in medical practice. Our object should be, not to dispute about what we think or believe—not what may, could, would, or should be, but what is; and this, I maintain, is only to be arrived at by making careful observations, and then tabulating the results. I trust, therefore, that physicians will assist me in the project of collecting cases of pneumonia, and tabulating them according to a uniform plan. Let us first obtain the facts, and learn how to read them afterwards. "It does not become me," says Dr. Barclay, "to offer any opposition to a praiseworthy effort, even though I am convinced it is labour thrown away." Now, it is maintained by some that no praiseworthy effort, if fairly tried, can ever be thrown away; and what can be more worthy of our regard than the desire to settle on some fixed basis the opposing and perplexing statements as to medical practice? Admitting the difficulty and the liability to error, it is certain that a united effort would do much. Difficulties may be overcome, errors corrected, if, instead of holding aloof, hospital and other physicians would set their clerks or assistants at work to tabulate cases on a uniform plan. In this manner it is my firm conviction that the treatment of pneumonia might be placed on as secure a basis as is the prevention of small-pox by vaccination. All we require is tabulated results; and if any member of the profession will co-operate with me in this effort I shall have great pleasure in forwarding to him a printed schedule, whereby, with little trouble to himself, he might greatly assist in forwarding so desirable a conclusion. In the meantime, I trust that the profession will not be induced to distrust too strongly medical statistics, but, whilst admitting their liability to error, make a strenuous effort, by a large experience, to place them on such a secure basis as shall advance our knowledge of the healing art.

APPENDIX OF CASES.

Out of the 129 cases tabulated I have selected 12 capable of illustrating, as it seems to me, the theory and practice inculcated in the preceding pages.

CASE I.*—*Pneumonia on left side—ushered in by Violent Vomiting and Gastric Pain—Convalescent in five days—Rapid recovery.*

HISTORY.—Edward Nugent, æt. 26, a waiter—admitted November 8th, 1858. Has always enjoyed good health until about three weeks ago, when he went to Liverpool from Glasgow by water, and suffered very severely from sea sickness. Three days afterwards, on the return passage, he was again very sick, and for a few days after felt soreness in the epigastric region. He then became quite well until Monday the 8th, at 1 P.M., when, whilst cleaning plate, and about ten minutes after eating a hearty dinner, he was suddenly seized with severe pain in the epigastrium, cold sweats, vertigo, desire to vomit, but inability to do so. He was immediately conveyed to the Infirmary.

SYMPTOMS ON ADMISSION.—The patient was pale and livid, almost pulseless, and complained of sickness, cold, profuse clammy perspiration, and great pain in epigastrium, increased on pressure. Shortly after admission he vomited what he had taken at dinner, but was not relieved; warm bottles were applied to his feet, and hot fomentations to the painful part. His suffering continued; at 4 P.M. six leeches were applied to the epigastrium, and ʒss of solution of Muriate of Morphia administered. These remedies gave some relief, and he remained in comparative ease till about 10 P.M., when some *Magn. Sulph.* was given, as the bowels had been costive for some days previously.

PROGRESS OF THE CASE.—*November 9th.*—He had no sleep during the night, and his symptoms have remained stationary. He has had three or four dark-coloured stools. Early in the morning he was ordered for the vomiting ℞ *Creasoti* gtt. ij; *Sol. Mur. Morph.* ʒss; *ft. haust.*; also a table-spoonful of port wine every hour. At the visit (noon) his symptoms had in no way abated, and he was ordered to *continue the*

* Reported by Mr. Arthur Cartington, Clinical Clerk.

wine; to take beef-tea in small quantities; and a tea-spoonful of the following mixture every hour until the pain decreased:—R Sol. Mur. Morph. ʒij; Sp. Æth. Sulph. ʒvj; Ft. mist. The mixture caused great relief, and in the afternoon he was able to bear further examination. The cardiac sounds were indistinct; pulse 58, extremely feeble and intermitting. Respiration laboured, and the pain in epigastrium increased during inspiration. There was slight harshness of inspiration, and increased vocal resonance under both clavicles. He had great pain at the back of his head, and some giddiness; tongue dry and furred; no appetite; great thirst; no perceptible swelling in epigastrium; abdomen tender and hot; urine natural in colour and quantity, but *only a slight trace of chlorides.* In the evening he was better, the pain had greatly subsided, and there was less sickness; he was able to retain some small quantities of beef-tea. Slight dulness, increase of vocal resonance, and crepitation, were detected at the base of the left lung posteriorly. *Nov.* 10th.—He passed a tolerably good night, and had some sleep; the epigastric pain and sickness still further diminished. Pulse 98, weak. The physical signs observed in left lung last evening were not audible at visit, but were again heard in the evening. *Ordered to discontinue the mixture, and to continue the wine and beef-tea in small quantities. Nov.* 11th.—He passed a good night; he still has slight sickness and tenderness over epigastrium. He complains of pain in the left breast, increased during inspiration; he has some shortness of breath, troublesome cough, and a greyish tenacious sputum containing a few rusty-coloured masses. Marked dulness, with increased vocal resonance, and clear crepitation, audible over lower third of left side posteriorly. Pulse 88, tolerably full; tongue loaded. The patient says he has had rigors every day since admission, and yesterday was so cold that he had warm bottles applied to his feet. On examination of the urine, the chlorides were still diminished, and there was a deposit of triple phosphates. *Nov.* 12th—Now sleeps well. His appetite is much improved. The epigastric pain and tenderness and the sickness have disappeared. Pulse 90, full and regular. Crepitation very fine; vocal resonance still increased. Cough not so bad, no rusty masses in the sputum. *Nov.* 13th—The crepitation has disappeared; there is some harshness of inspiration. Sputum muco-purulent. Chlorides abundant in the urine. *Convalescent.* His bowels being confined, *he was ordered an enema of warm water. Nov.* 15th.—Respiration quite natural. He says he only feels a little weak, but is otherwise so well that he insists on being discharged.

Commentary.—In this case of severe gastric irritation, pneumonia came on in the Infirmary—was well characterised by all the symptoms and physical signs of the disease, was limited to the posterior third of the left lung, occurred in a healthy young man, and was treated by stimulants and nutrients from the beginning.

The result was recovery on the fifth day and discharge from the hospital at his own request quite well on the seventh day. It is the most rapid recovery from decided pneumonia that has ever fallen under my notice. The facts of this case are also entirely opposed to the notions of those who consider that inflammation is in some way connected with a sthenic or excited state of the system. The man was in perfect health when seized with the gastric spasms, and was by them reduced to a pulseless and exceedingly prostrated state, with cold clammy sweats. It was in this weakened condition that the pneumonia arose, and its limited extent and short course I ascribe to the stimulants, nutrients, and quietude with which it was treated from the first.

CASE II.*—*Pneumonia on Right Side and slight Pleuritis—Convalescent in twelve days—Rapid recovery.*

HISTORY.—Roderick M'Farlane, æt. 20, a gardener of healthy and robust constitution—admitted December 17th, 1856. On the 19th instant felt unwell, with a sensation of cold in the back. On the 13th had pain in the right infra-axillary region, increased on deep inspiration, with hot skin, headache, thirst, and loss of appetite, symptoms which have continued ever since. On the 14th, cough appeared with scanty expectoration. Has taken a dose of castor-oil and some pills.

SYMPTOMS ON ADMISSION.—Expansion on both sides of chest equal. Respirations twenty-four in the minute, not laboured. Can lie on either side, but prefers lying on the back. Pain during deep inspiration over right infra-axillary region ; slight cough ; scanty expectoration—frothy and mucous. On percussion, cracked-pot resonance extends from clavicle to fifth rib on right side. Below this level percussion is dull. There is also decided dulness posteriorly from spine of scapula to base. Elsewhere percussion natural. On auscultation, puerile respiration over left front ; over right front superiorly respiration is harsh, without rale ; below fifth rib it is suppressed. Posteriorly, over two lower thirds, double friction is audible, with fine crepitation at the close of inspiration ; on left side occasional sibilus, with a few moist rattles at close of inspiration over lower third. The vocal resonance is increased and sharp on right side anteriorly, but greatly increased and ægophonic posteriorly over area of dulness. Pulse 104, incompressible and full. Skin hot and dry. Tongue in centre brown, dry, and cracked ; edges moist and clean. No appetite ; great thirst ; bowels always regular, but have been opened by laxatives. Urine natural. Other functions normal. R. Sol. Antim. Tart. ℥ss ; Aquæ Ammon. Acet. ℥j ; Aquæ ℥viss. M. Habeat sextam partem quartâ quâque horâ.

* Reported by Dr. J. Glen, Resident Clinical Physician.

PROGRESS OF THE CASE.—*December* 18*th*.—Grazing friction audible over the right infra-mammary region. Crepitation distinct over right back inferiorly. Pulse 120, soft. Sputum scanty, consisting of orange-coloured, gelatinous masses. Otherwise the same. *Dec.* 20*th*.—Crepitations very coarse over right back. Fever abated, tongue moist and clean. Pulse 72, of good strength. Temperature of skin natural. *Omitt. mist. Dec.* 22*d*.—Crepitation and friction disappeared from right back. Abundant sediment of lithates in the urine. ℞ *Sp. Æther. Nit.* ʒiij; *Vin. Sem. Colchici*, ʒj; *Aquam ad* ℥vj. *M. Two table-spoonfuls to be taken every four hours. Dec.* 24*th*.—Dulness over right back and cracked-pot sound anteriorly greatly diminished. For the last three days has had profuse diaphoresis. Urine again natural. Convalescent. *Omitt. mist.* To have steak diet. *Dec.* 26*th*.—No dulness anywhere; respirations natural. Is quite recovered; but as the weather was severe, and he had to work immediately in the open air, if dismissed, he was not discharged until January 2d.

Commentary.—This young man was first seized with illness on the 12th of December, and was admitted on the 17th, when hepatisation of the lung was found to have occurred in the lower two-thirds of the organ on the right side, combined with slight pleuritis. Fever was well marked, the pulse full and incompressible. On the 22d the exudation was thoroughly softened and passing off from the economy principally by the urine, but partly by the skin. On the 24th, twelve days after the commencement of the disease, all the symptoms had disappeared, and he commenced to take beef-steak. On the 26th all trace of the disease had disappeared. The treatment consisted at first of slight salines and rest, then of a diuretic mixture to favour excretion of the effete products by the urine, and lastly of steak diet. From the first commencement to the complete disappearance of the disease was fourteen days; to the abatement of fever and commencing resolution, eight days; and to convalescence, twelve days. The febrile phenomena in this case were unusually well pronounced. The pulse was full and incompressible—in fact, hard; the skin hot and dry. Tongue furred and dry; no appetite; great thirst, etc. In short, this young vigorous lad presented all those symptoms in which we are instructed by most writers to bleed, and in which it has been argued, that without bleeding a fatal suppuration was likely to occur. I need scarcely add, that the propriety of such practice, as well as the probable fatality, were alike negatived by the result.

Case III.*—*Pneumonia on the Right Side—Early and repeated Venesection—Convalescent in fourteen days—Slow Recovery.*

History.—James M'Quair, tailor, æt. 29.—admitted June 4th, 1865. This man has been of intemperate habits during the last five years. On the 26th of May, after severe drinking and exertion, followed by exposure to the night air, he was attacked early in the morning with rigor, chilliness, a feeling of weight over his whole body, and a dull heavy pain in the right chest. He drank several glasses of whisky and water to allay his thirst, and kept his bed, occasionally vomiting, and going out of doors to stool, until the 30th. He now felt very feverish, weak, and unwell, and a soup-plateful of blood was extracted from the arm (ʒxxiv). Venesection to the same amount was made on the following day; but the pains in the side, with sanguineous cough and expectoration continuing, he came to the Infirmary.

Symptoms on Admission.—On admission, the patient has an anxious and flushed appearance, and feels very weak. The respiration is hurried, 42 in a minute, and the lower part of the right lung expands little. Cough is short, frequent, and suppressed; the expectoration scanty, consisting of gelatinous mucus slightly tinged with blood. On percussion, there is marked comparative dulness over the inferior half of the right lung, but the upper half anteriorly, especially at the apex, though flat in tone, gives out a tympanitic and somewhat intestinal note. On auscultation, crepitation is audible all over the right lung, both anteriorly and posteriorly, and the vocal resonance is much increased over the dull portion. The left lung is normal. The pulse is 100, hard and incompressible. Heart normal. Tongue dry, and covered with a dark-brown fur, and the teeth surrounded by sordes. Appetite gone; great thirst; the vomiting, which existed at the commencement of the attack, has now ceased. Abdominal viscera normal; bowels regular. Skin dry and hot to the feel. Urine high-coloured and diminished in quantity, clear and without sediment. No trace of chlorides; no albumen. Nervous system normal. ℞ Antim. Tart. gr. iij; Aquæ ʒvj; Solve. One ounce to be taken every three hours.

Progress of the Case.—*June 5th.*—Says he feels better; pulse 90, full and compressible, but in the evening it fell to 80, and became soft. *June 8th.*—Pulse 78, soft, breathing more easy. On percussion, the lower half of right lung is dull, but the upper half is resonant, with distinct cracked-pot sound. Fine crepitation audible over the whole of right chest. *June 8th.*—The whole of the right lung in front has become resonant on percussion; otherwise the same. Faint trace of chlorides in the urine. *June 9th.*—Chlorides abundant in the urine. *June 10th.*—Percussion resonant and equal over both sides of chest anteriorly. Under right clavicle, cracked-pot sound still audible. Crepitation much less inferiorly, but continues at the apex, with increase of

* Reported by Mr. Robert Byers, Clinical Clerk.

vocal resonance. Posteriorly, percussion over right lung dull inferiorly, with loud crepitation and ægophonic resonance of voice. The patient feels much better, though weak. Respiration free. Pulse 72, soft and regular. Considerable diaphoresis. Urine deposits on cooling a large amount of lithates. Convalescent. ℞ Antim. Tart. gr. ij ; Tinct. Camph. ca. 5ij ; Decoct. Serpent. 5xij. M. 5j. to be taken every three hours. June 14th.— Physical signs of right lung, with the exception of cracked-put sound, much diminished. Has been taking, during the last three days, seuk diet, with 5iv of wine. From this time he improved slowly, the crepitation and dulness posteriorly gradually disappeared, but the cracked-pot sound continued with great intensity up to the 20th of June. His strength was not sufficient to admit of his discharge until the 3d of July.

Commentary.—This was a case in which nearly the whole of the right lung became pneumonic, and where we had an opportunity of convincing ourselves that full and repeated bleeding, although practised so early as the second and third days, had no beneficial influence on the progress of the disease. It should also be remarked, that these bleedings were practised in accordance with the rules laid down in systematic writings—that is to say, not only early, but when the pulse was accelerated, hard, and incompressible, with all the characteristic symptoms of the disease. Surely, if bleedings could cut short or diminish the duration of a pneumonia, it might have been expected in this case. Yet so far from proving beneficial, they appear to me to have assisted in prolonging the case, and preventing resolution and recovery. For although the critical diaphoresis, and discharge of lithates by urine, occurred on the fourteenth day, the subsequent weakness was considerable, and the convalescence prolonged to the thirty-seventh day.

CASE IV.*—*Erysipelas of the Face followed by Pneumonia of the Right Side—Convalescent in seven days—Rapid recovery.*

HISTORY.—Margaret Armstrong, æt. 28, wife of a shoemaker, of robust healthy appearance—admitted December 7, 1855. She states that she was quite well up to Wednesday evening last (December 5th), when, after being engaged for some time in washing, she was seized with rigors and febrile symptoms. Next morning her face felt painful and swollen, and has continued so up to the time of admission. When examined in the ward, the whole of the face and forehead was of a fiery red colour, the integuments, and especially the eyelids, greatly swollen, with a few bullæ on each cheek, full of yellow lymph ; the skin every-

─────────────────────────────
* Reported by Mr. G. Robertson, Clinical Clerk.

where hot, and in the face giving rise to a severe smarting sensation. Tongue and lips dry, covered with black sordes ; great thirst ; no appetite ; cephalagia ; pulse 130, soft ; bowels not open.   Urine natural in quantity, turbid from pinkish sediment, containing a considerable amount of albumen and a very scanty quantity of chlorides.   *To have 3ss of castor oil, and the face to be covered with cloths wrung out of warm water.*

PROGRESS OF THE CASE.—*December 11th.*—To-day the face is assuming its natural colour, the epidermis desquamating.   There is no albumen in the urine, and the chlorides are abundant.   *Dec. 13th.*— The erysipelas has now disappeared, but there is a general aspect of prostration.   She has had a short cough for the last two days, which cannot be ascertained to have been ushered in by rigors.   Breathing hurried and laborious.   Pulse 92, small.   On percussing the chest posteriorly, there is comparative dulness over right back inferiorly.   On auscultation, a fine crepitation is audible there on inspiration, with sonorous and sibilant rales and increased resonance (almost pealing) of the voice.   Dry rales are also heard anteriorly on this side, with expiration and inferiorly coarse moist rale.   There is no expectoration. Urine abundant, of brick-dust colour, which disappears on the addition of heat ; sp. gr. 1022, no albumen, and the chlorides have disappeared. *To have beef-tea, and 3vj of wine daily.   Dec. 17th.*—The pneumonia, since last report, has produced complete dulness, with bronchophony in the lower third of right lung, which is, however, now disappearing. There have been all the usual symptoms, with gelatinous rusty sputa. To-day, chlorides in urine are more abundant.   *Dec. 19th.*—Diseased lung more resonant on percussion.   Breathing more natural, free from moist rale.   Still increase of vocal resonance.   Chlorides abundant in urine.   Convalescent.   *Diminish wine to 3iij daily.   Dec. 24th.*—To-day can breathe without difficulty ; respiration on right side normal, but still some increase of vocal resonance ; pulse 60, of good strength. Expresses herself as being quite well.   Has been for the last two days on steak diet, and walking about the ward.   Wishes to leave the hospital. Dismissed.

Commentary.—The erysipelas in this case was very severe, but occurring, as it did, in a healthy young woman, gave us little concern, and was allowed to take its natural course.   Warm water applications only were employed to relieve the smarting.   The disease, in consequence, had disappeared by the seventh day.   The chlorides in the urine were diminished during the accession of the fever and presence of the eruption, and returned abundantly when the erysipelas had disappeared.   The ward at this time was very cold, from some of the ventilators, which allowed the admission of frosty air, not having been closed.   Pneumonia on one side came on, and the chlorides again disappeared from the urine. The attack, supervening on an acute febrile disease, was characterised by great prostration of the system and weak pulse throughout. But, under the careful exhibition of nutrients and six ounces of wine daily, she made a rapid recovery. The pneumonia was detected on the 13th. The chlorides had returned on the 19th, when she became convalescent, and she was dismissed at her own request, quite well, on the 24th.

CASE V.*—*Double Pneumonia—Great Dyspnœa—No Bleeding—Local Warmth and Restoratives—Convalescent in eleven days—Rapid Recovery.*

HISTORY.—Peter Robertson, æt. 51, a tolerably robust man, house-painter—admitted May 11, 1857. On Tuesday last, the 5th instant, when washing the outside of a house, he got wet through from the dripping of water. In the evening had a rigor, which continued more or less all night. On the following morning had a short cough, and a thick yellow sputum. These symptoms continued the two following days, with pain in the left breast anteriorly; but he continued at his work, although feeling very weak. On the 9th he was obliged to go to bed, and observed his sputum to be tinged with blood. Yesterday again had rigors, with cramps in the arms and elbows.

SYMPTOMS ON ADMISSION.—On percussion there is marked dulness over the lower two-thirds of the left lung posteriorly, with tubular breathing and coarse mucous rale on inspiration. The vocal resonance is ægophonic inferiorly, and bronchophonic over the middle third. Right side and anterior surfaces normal. Sputum copious and viscid, mixed with dark blood. Pulse 100, small and weak. Respirations 36 per minute. Skin moist. Other functions normal. ℞ Liq. Ammon. Acet. ℨj; Sp. Æther. Nitric. ℨss; Vin. Antim. ℨiss; Aquam ad ℥vj. M. One table-spoonful to be taken every three hours.

PROGRESS OF THE CASE.—May 12th—Dulness on percussion over lower third of right back, in addition to that on the left, with tubular breathing and increased vocal resonance. Physical signs otherwise the same. Respirations are 40 in the minute, laborious and catching. Sputum gelatinous and rusty. Pulse 120, weak. Face livid, and expressive of great anxiety. Urine high coloured, scanty, and deficient in chlorides. Warm fomentations to be applied over left side, and to have ℨiv of wine. May 13th—Much better. Respiration easy. No lividity or anxiety of countenance. Cough diminished. Pulse 80, soft, but of good strength. Omit mist. Nutrients. May 14th—Less dulness and crepitation on left side; on right side crepitation fully established. Chlorides present to a slight degree in urine, and urates abundant

---

* Reported by Mr. W. H. Davies, Clinical Clerk.

Pulse 74, regular. Appetite returning. Tongue clean. *Steak diet.*
May 16th.—Is now convalescent. Urine natural. Percussion resonant
over both backs ; inspiratory murmurs heard, but no moist rales. Cough
painless. Still gelatinous sputum without blood. Has been out of
bed, and feels tolerably strong. *May 19th.*—Has been up all day, and
says he is quite well. *May 20th.*—Dismissed.

Commentary.—This was a severe case of double pneumonia,
with great dyspnœa, impending suffocation, and great weakness on
the seventh day of the disease, when wine was administered. On
the following day he was better, and continued to improve, so that on
the fifth day after admission he was fully convalescent, and on the
ninth was quite well and returned to his work. I never saw a case
in which the symptoms were more urgent than in this man the day
after his admission, and in which the livid and anxious countenance,
the intense dyspnœa, the bloody sputum and feeble pulse, gave
stronger evidence of impending dissolution. A question arises
whether, if this man had been bled, he would have been relieved.
I think this is very probable. But it appeared to me at the time,
that, considering the great prostration and weakness of the pulse,
the practice would have been fatal. Certain it is, that by following
an opposite treatment of warm fomentations locally, with wine and
nutrients internally, these symptoms quickly subsided, and next
day he was found breathing easily ; and from that moment, though
both lungs were affected, speedily recovered. (See also Case VII.)
In a similar case, recently published by Dr. Markham, a bleeding
of ℥vj caused marked and immediate relief, and on this ground
the practice of bleeding in such cases is again inculcated. Now,
much will depend upon the character of the pulse and amount of
exhaustion—two points not referred to by Dr. Markham. It is to
be observed, however, that whilst the above case, with the same
impending dissolution from asphyxia and double pneumonia, was
convalescent in five days after entering the house, and left the
hospital quite well on the ninth day, Dr. Markham's case, though
relieved by bleeding, had a long convalescence, with pericarditis
and pleuritic abscess.* In the same manner, it will be seen on reference to Case VIII., in which the practice of early venesection was
followed, a prolonged convalescence was also the result.

* British Med. Journal, Feb. 4, 1865.

CASE VI.*—*Double Pneumonia, with urgent Symptoms, and full
strong Pulse—Pleuritis on Left Side—Five ounces of Blood
removed by Cupping—Convalescent in nine days—Recovery de-
layed in consequence of an attack of Acute Rheumatism.*

HISTORY.—John M'Farlane, æt. 30, a railway labourer—admitted
Nov. 12, 1856. Has been subject to a slight cough and expectoration,
sometimes tinged with blood, for the last ten winters; otherwise he has
enjoyed good health. On Nov. 9th, whilst working on a railway bank,
which was much exposed to wind and cold, he was suddenly seized with
great pain in his lower extremities; he, however, continued at his work
till the evening, when he experienced a sharp pain in his left side, with
difficulty of breathing and general febrile symptoms. He went to bed,
and on the 10th, feeling no better, he sent for a medical man, who
ordered a blister to be applied to the left side; he also gave him a
powder, and a mixture which made him very sick. The pain was
slightly relieved after the application of the blister, and he felt much
easier on the 11th, but on the 12th the pain increased, while the difficulty of breathing and of expectorating became so bad that he was
brought into the Infirmary.

SYMPTOMS ON ADMISSION.—His face was much flushed; skin hot
and dry; tongue moist, and with a white fur; great thirst; pulse 95,
full and regular; urine orange-coloured, with a copious sediment of
urates, only a slight trace of chlorides, and a trace of albumen. His
respirations were quick and laboured. Expectoration very tenacious,
with numerous rusty-coloured masses in it. Cough frequent and painful.
On the left side anteriorly percussion was good, but crepitation was
heard all over the front, with the exception of a space 2½ inches below
the clavicle, where the respiratory sounds were very harsh. Posteriorly
on this side there was marked dulness from the spine of the scapula to
the base of the lung, over which space loud crepitation was heard, and
pealing vocal resonance, more especially about the centre of the lung.
On the right side anteriorly there was slight comparative dulness over
a space extending from the clavicle two inches downwards. Posteriorly
on this side there was slight comparative dulness at apex, where expiration was prolonged, and the inspiratory murmur harsh. R Pulv. Doveri,
gr. x, to be taken immediately. R Sol. Antim. 3j ; Potass. Acet. 3ss; Aquam
ad 3viij ; ft. mist. Two table-spoonfuls every four hours.

PROGRESS OF THE CASE.—Nov. 13th.—Passed a sleepless night.
Cough incessant, and dyspnœa urgent; face livid. Pulse 112, full and
strong; sputum very copious, rusty and gelatinous. In addition to
physical signs formerly reported, there was faint crepitation all over
right back posteriorly (most distinct at apex), but no great increase of
vocal resonance; friction over left side anteriorly below nipple, both
with expiration and inspiration, but loudest with former, and posteriorly

* Reported by Mr. Arthur Garrington, Clinical Clerk.

marked dulness over inferior two-thirds, with loud crepitation and bron-chophony. *Ordered to be cupped to ʒv over region of pain on left side, and to take only one table-spoonful of the mixture, to which is to be added Sp. Æth. Nitr. ʒij. To have strong beef-tea and milk. Nov. 14th.*—Patient says he felt relieved by the cupping for 3 or 4 hours, but the pain re-turned afterwards as bad as before. There is still great dyspnœa and lividity of face ; expectorates about 18 oz. of purulent, gelatinous, frothy matter, tinged with rusty-coloured blood, during the 24 hours. Pulse 98, soft and irregular. *To have a table-spoonful of wine every hour. Omit mixture. Nov. 15th.*—Dyspnœa and pain in side much diminished. Sputum less rusty. Pulse 100, strong and regular. Very coarse crepi-tation (amounting to mucous rattles) heard over left side anteriorly. Respiratory murmurs harsh and dry over right side anteriorly. There is still marked comparative dulness over left back, and also in upper third of right back. Tubular breathing over upper fourth of right back, harsh inferiorly. Crepitation over left back, but more feeble than before. Vocal resonance the same. Urine quite clear, and no deposit. Chlorides have been increasing since the 13th, but are not yet in normal proportion. Still thirsty and feverish. ℞ *Sp. Æth. Nitr.* ʒiij ; *Potass. Acet.* ʒss ; *Aquam ad* ʒvj ; *ft. mist. To be taken as before. To continue the milk, wine, etc., and to have 6 oz. beef-steak. Nov. 18th.*—Patient says he feels very much better. All crepitation gone, but there is slightly increased vocal resonance on left side. Urine loaded with urates. *Con-valescent, but steak to be increased to 8 oz., and wine to be diminished to* ʒiv *daily. Nov. 24th.*—Has been getting gradually stronger since last re-port. Yesterday he got up for some time, walked about the ward, and exposed himself to draughts in the passages. This led to an attack of acute rheumatism, for which he was again confined to bed, and ordered Potass. Bicarb. ʒj three times a day. He gradually got better, and was quite free from muscular pains on Dec. 4th ; he got up on the 7th, and with the exception of slight weakness, felt quite well. 2 oz. extra beef-steak were ordered on the 11th, and he left the Infirmary on the 13th in perfect health.

Commentary.—This is what some former writers would have called an "exquisite" case of pneumonia, occurring in a man who, with some emphysema, was accustomed to have attacks of bronchitis and bloody expectoration every winter. It presented all the symptoms of the disease, including pain in the side, great dyspnœa, lividity of the face, strong and full pulse, with copious rusty sputa. Physical signs also proved it to consist of hepatisation of the two inferior thirds of the left lung, and of the superior half of the right lung. Occurring in the year 1858, it disposes of two theo-retical statements which have of late been much discussed—viz. 1st, That such cases are now not to be met with ; and, 2d, that if they should occur, bleeding would again be required for their treatment. In this respect the case resembles that of Roderick M'Farlane, Case II.; and in severity that of Peter Robertson, Case IV. In consequence of the dyspnœa and evident engorgement of the right side of the heart, he was cupped, and 5v of blood extracted, with the effect of relieving his symptoms, but for a time only, as they returned with equal intensity in a few hours. This is the result which usually followed large venesections, and which misled practitioners as to their utility. I have no doubt that a large bleeding in this case, if it had not proved fatal, would have seriously prolonged his recovery, which commenced under an opposite treatment on the ninth day. The case inculcates another caution—viz. the necessity of avoiding exposure to cold during convalescence, as in the debilitated condition which then exists there is very likely to be a relapse, or some other form of febrile disease, again proving that these are the results of weakness rather than of strength.

CASE VII.*—*Double Pneumonia, involving the whole of the Right Lung, and the lower two-thirds of the Left Lung—Cardiac disease—No Bleeding—Palliative effect of warm poultices——Convalescent in fourteen days—Dismissed well from the Infirmary after sixteen days' Residence.*

HISTORY.—John Baker, æt. 57, hawker—admitted December 30, 1860. This man was discharged from the army in 1847 in consequence of long-standing chest-disease, attended with cough, expectoration, hæmoptysis, and aphonia. Nine years ago he had severe rheumatism, since which time he has been subject to palpitations. On the evening of the 14th, after exposure to inclement weather, he was seized with a severe rigor, followed by intense febrile symptoms, cough, and expectoration. On the 16th he felt pain at the base of right lung anteriorly. These symptoms increased until he was admitted into the Infirmary.

SYMPTOMS ON ADMISSION.—Urgent dyspnœa, respirations being 56 in the minute. A cutting pain in the right chest anteriorly, increased on inspiration. Occasionally severe cough, with scanty frothy expectoration. On percussion, the anterior surface of the chest is resonant, with the exception of the lower third of the right lung, over which there is dulness. On auscultation there is crepitation heard over the dull portion on the right side, and great harshness of breathing in the upper two-thirds. Posteriorly there is dulness on percussion over the lower two-thirds of the right lung, with crepitation, sibilation on expiration,

---

* Reported by Mr. Archibald Hamilton, Clinical Clerk.

and great increase of vocal resonance on auscultation. On the left side there was no dulness on percussion, but slight crepitation at the base on auscultation. Pulse 104, of fair strength. Heart not examined, in consequence of the great dyspnœa ; slight headache ; tongue covered with a white moist fur ; great thirst ; no appetite ; bowels open ; face flushed ; eyes suffused ; skin hot, but not dry. Urine sp. gr. 1025, high-coloured, clear, no albumen, chlorides diminished. ℞ Liq. Acetat. Ammon. ʒj ; Sp. Æther. Nit. ʒij ; Aquæ ʒv. M. A table-spoonful to be taken every four hours. To have strong beef-tea.

PROGRESS OF THE CASE.—December 21st.—Passed a restless night. Intensity of the symptoms not diminished. On percussion over the back, dulness on the right side now extends from the apex to the base, and over the lower third of the lung on the left side. On auscultation, tubular breathing, crepitation, and ægophony very distinct on the right side, and loud crepitation over the dull portion on the left side. Above on this side respiration puerile. Pulse 98, of fair strength. The great dyspnœa and harsh respiration renders examination of the heart unsatisfactory ; but on asking him to hold his breath for a moment, a distinct blowing murmur is heard with the first sound at the apex. Strong headache. Great pain in right side. Chlorides in clear urine further diminished. A warm poultice to be put over lower half of right chest. Continue beef-tea. Dec. 22d.—All the urgent symptoms continue, with the exception of the pain on right side, which is now gone, and replaced by pain on left side. Expectoration gelatinous, rusty, interspersed with orange-coloured masses. Urine loaded with lithates. Omit Saline Mixture ; ℞ Sp. Æther. Nit. ʒiij ; Vin. Sem. Colch. ʒj ; Aquæ ʒvss. M. Ft. mist. Two table-spoonfuls to be taken every four hours. A large warm poultice over the left chest. Dec. 23d.—Was found last evening at the visit to be breathing tranquilly ; free from pain ; respirations 44 in the minute ; pulse 104, soft ; has taken ʒj of wine in water. Experienced great relief from the warm poultices. To-day, at the visit, still slight pain on coughing ; sputa orange-coloured ; dulness diminished on right side, but occupies two lower thirds of the left lung. Urine densely loaded with lithates. To have ʒiv of port wine daily. Dec. 25th.—Urine still loaded with lithates. The chlorides have returned. Pulse 80, soft. Dec. 28th.—Slept well. Tongue moist, clean at the edges. Pulse 76, soft. Physical signs diminished in intensity, but crepitation still audible distantly over diseased lungs. Had ʒiv of steak for dinner, which he ate with relish. Convalescent. January 4th.—Since last report the symptoms and physical signs have rapidly disappeared, with the exception of slight dulness and increased vocal resonance at the base of left lung. Blowing murmur at cardiac apex very soft. Dismissed.

Commentary.—This was perhaps the most severe and most extensive case of pneumonia I ever saw, involving, as it did, the whole of the right and two-thirds of the left lung. It was also associated with mitral incompetency of the heart, and occasioned an amount of dyspnœa, lividity of the face, pain, and general uneasiness seldom witnessed. Having satisfied myself, however, from previous cases, that the danger of these symptoms is more apparent than real, I did not attempt even to alleviate them by cupping, as was done in the last case. I applied large warm poultices over the painful sides, which at once caused great relief, and appeared to be both more soothing to the patient and more permanent in its effect than small bleedings. (See also Case V.) Since the occurrence of this case I have continued the practice with the best results, and have never employed blood-letting even as a palliative—not that I think the loss of a small quantity of blood dangerous, or incapable of giving relief, but that it is unnecessary. Large warm poultices relieve more, and may possibly serve to assist the transformation of the exudation in the lung, and facilitate recovery.

CASE VIII.*—*Double Pneumonia, involving the whole of the Right Side and one-third of the Left Side—Albuminuria—bled on the day of Attack—great Prostration—convalescent on the twenty-seventh day, and could only be dismissed from the Infirmary on the thirty-eighth day.*

HISTORY.—James Potter, æt. 47, quarryman—admitted into the clinical ward of the Royal Infirmary, December 19, 1860. He says he has always been robust, but not of very temperate habits. During the last eight years has had two or three severe attacks of inflammation in the chest, similar to that he now labours under. On the 17th instant, when working in a tunnel, with wet clothes on and exposed to a strong current of wind, he was seized with a rigor, headache, and thirst. He returned home at half-past five, but could take no nourishment, and then experienced pain in his right side. This increased so rapidly that he sent for a medical man, who took 5xx of blood from his right arm by venesection, remarking, at the same time, that it was not customary to bleed nowadays. The patient thinks he got relief for a short time after the operation; but during the night he was very restless, and had great thirst, severe headache, hot skin, pain in the side, and cough. On the following day all his symptoms were aggravated, and he commenced to expectorate. In the evening he was ordered to take a sweating powder and an ounce of Epsom salts; but finding himself worse next morning, entered the Infirmary about 1 P.M.

SYMPTOMS ON ADMISSION.—Though in a state of great exhaustion, could walk and give a clear account of his case. He was, however,

* Reported by Mr. Peter M. Braidwood, Clinical Clerk.

immediately put to bed, and ordered two table-spoonfuls of port wine in strong beef-tea to be taken every two or three hours, while his examination was postponed until the evening visit. *Vespere, 9 p.m.*—The patient had a short frequent cough, with expectoration, which was frothy, tenacious, and slightly rusty. Complains of soreness in the right infra-mammary region, which becomes pain on coughing, taking a long breath, or making any exertion. Breathing short and hurried—expiration prolonged. On percussion anteriorly, there is dulness over the whole of right chest, but more marked from a horizontal line drawn an inch above the nipple, down to the hepatic dulness. Left lung resonant. On auscultation there is crepitation over the whole right side of chest from apex to base, but loudest about two inches above the nipple. There is also great increase of the vocal resonance. On the left side breathing is puerile. Posteriorly complete dulness, with crepitation and pealing resonance of the voice over the two lower thirds of the right lung, with tubular breathing over the upper third. Left side respiration everywhere puerile. Pulse 106, weak. Lips dry. Tongue furred in the centre, moist at the edges. Disagreeable taste in the mouth. No appetite. Has had two stools since admission. Frontal headache, with horrible dreams at night, which are broken by frequent cough. Urine of a muddy orange colour, sp. gr. 1015. Chlorides greatly diminished, but a considerable amount of albumen present. Skin hot but slightly moist. Patient could only lie on the back, and seemed greatly prostrated.

PROGRESS OF THE CASE.—*December 20th.*—Slept well last night. The breathing easier. Expectoration profuse, consisting of tenacious gelatinous matter of the colour of green-gage juice. Marked dulness over the whole right lung, with tubular breathing over the upper third. The physical signs and other symptoms the same. *To have ʒvj of wine.* ℞ *Vin. Antim.* ʒj ; *Sol. Ammon. Acet.* ʒj ; *Aquæ* ʒv. *M. A table-spoonful every four hours. Dec. 21st.*—Yesterday evening the house physician detected crepitation over lower third of right back. Passed a restless night. To-day is greatly exhausted, cannot move, face pale and pinched. Breathing loud and tracheal ; respirations 48 per minute ; expectoration more scanty but of the same character. Cardiac sounds indistinct. Pulse 88, weak, irregular, and intermittent. Constant tendency to sleep. Urine still albuminous, with scanty chlorides. In consequence of his extreme exhaustion, the chest was not examined physically. *To have a table-spoonful of port wine in beef-tea every two hours. Dec. 22d.*—Yesterday afternoon the bowels were well opened. Slept little during the night, being harassed with cough, dyspnœa, and frightful dreams. To-day there is dulness, tubular breathing, and broncho-phony below the left scapula. On the right side physical signs unchanged. No appetite, but takes the nutrients regularly. *Omit mixture. Dec. 23d.*—Restless night, but somewhat better to-day. The tubular breathing over the upper third of right lung and under the left scapula now transformed into coarse crepitation. Still great exhaustion. *Dec. 24th.*—Passed a better night. Pulse 84, fuller, and less irregular.

Breathing easier and less rapid. Expectoration less tenacious, but frothy, of dirty yellow colour. *Dec. 31st.*—Has been much the same since last report. Thirst and febrile symptoms continue—especially at night. Has little appetite, but ordered to try a steak diet. *January 13th.*—Since last report he has been very gradually gaining strength. The vocal resonance, tubular breathing, and crepitation on both sides of the chest posteriorly still continue, but are now much diminished. Expectoration small in quantity, frothy, mucous, and slightly purulent. Slept well last night, and had less febrile excitement. Pulse 78, of good strength. He could only to-day be declared convalescent. *Jan. 26th.*—Strength has been slowly improving. There is still slight cough and expectoration. Urine continues albuminous. For the last few days has been taking exercise in the open air. Dismissed.

April 28th.—He was re-admitted, saying that since his dismissal he has been working in a tunnel near Peebles. Three days ago he was seized with shivering, but worked on for three hours. He then went home, and sent for a medical man who cupped him, but he does not know how much blood he lost, as he became unconscious. On admission there was dulness over the whole right lung anteriorly, most marked from the apex to the third rib. On auscultation there was tubular breathing over the upper third, and crepitation over the lower two-thirds of the lung, with coarse double friction murmur and increased vocal resonance. On the left side anteriorly, there is dulness from the apex down to the fourth rib, below which percussion was resonant. On auscultation tubular breathing with sibilation on inspiration and increased vocal resonance. Posteriorly on right side marked dulness from the apex to lower angle of scapula, and on the left side from apex to base. Over the whole of the dull portion breathing is tubular, with double friction on the right side, and crepitation at the base on the left side. Cough severe ; great dyspnœa ; expectoration moderate, gelatinous, and of a dirty green colour. Prostration extreme. Pulse 108, very weak.

He was treated in the same manner as during the former attack. On the 16th of May he was convalescent, though still very weak, and readily took an egg and rice pudding for dinner. He has had ℥vj of port wine daily. From this he slowly recovered, and was dismissed May 30th, with dulness on percussion over right lung from apex to the lower angle of scapula ; but, with the exception of harshness on inspiration over the dull portion, otherwise in a normal state.

Commentary.—This man, attacked with acute pneumonia, was bled on the very day of the attack, but the operation, instead of producing any benefit, was followed by such extreme prostration, that his dissolution was hourly expected for three days. Beef-tea with wine were assiduously administered, and he slowly rallied. Convalescence could not be said to have fairly set in until the twenty-seventh day of the disease, and he could not be discharged from the Infirmary until the thirty-eighth day.

What a remarkable contrast do the last two cases present; and their careful study will, I think, dispose of many questions which have been recently agitated as to the treatment of pneumonia. Both cases were those of men whose previous health had been deteriorated by long-standing disease. They both occurred exactly at the same time, and lay in the clinical ward together. The advantage of age and of constitutional vigour was on the side of Potter. Both had double pneumonia, but in Potter it was not so extensive as in Baker. Both had complications, but that of Baker was the one most liable to intensify a pulmonary disease. Thus in both these extreme cases the actual advantages were all on the side of Potter. Notwithstanding, his prostration was extreme, and recovery prolonged, whilst the other rallied rapidly, and soon regained his strength. All experience tends to prove that the cause of this difference was entirely dependent on the treatment. The venesection, though practised on the very day of the attack—that is, when we are told by systematic writers it is capable of producing the best effects—caused a prostration that was nearly fatal. It is also to be observed that in the second attack he was cupped to syncope, with a like prostrating result.

Neither did the bleeding, whether by venesection or cupping, produce that marked relief or palliation of the symptoms which has recently been so strongly contended for. On the contrary, it may frequently be observed how very temporary such relief occasioned by bleeding often is, whereas in the case of Baker large warm poultices were of much greater value. On the whole, if the study of individual cases is likely to impress us with the advantage of treatment, I would confidently recommend a study of the 4 severe cases of double pneumonia now recorded. But further, my Statistical Table distinctly shows that of 15 cases where the whole of one lung was involved, and in 26 cases where portions of both lungs were affected, the rapidity of recovery was not so much dependent, as is generally supposed, on the extent of tissue involved, as on the restorative or weakening systems of treatment employed.

CASE IX.*—*Double Pneumonia—Treatment by Mercury, which caused Profuse Salivation before Admission—Prolonged Recovery.*

HISTORY.—Robert Jude, æt. 36, a bricklayer—admitted 10th December 1855. On the 1st instant, while engaged building bricks round a boiler, the weather being very cold and windy, he suddenly felt a pain in the chest, deep-seated, half way between the ensiform cartilage and umbilicus. The pain rapidly grew worse, and caused nausea, but he could not vomit. He immediately went home, took some gruel, and went to bed. On the 4th, a medical man gave him some pills, one of which he took every third hour. On the 6th his teeth were loose, the gums very tender, and the tongue swollen to twice its natural size, so that he could not spit out the excessive amount of saliva that was secreted, and which consequently flowed from his mouth. He also had pain in the loins.

SYMPTOMS ON ADMISSION.—On admission the excessive salivation has much diminished, but there is still tenderness and redness of the gums, with considerable discharge from the mouth. The breath fœtid, the tongue covered with a dense dirty white coating. The bowels, while taking the pills, were open from six to seven times a-day ; they are now regular. His diet has been confined to farinaceous articles. On percussing the chest anteriorly, it is everywhere resonant, but posteriorly it is dull on both sides, most so on left side. On auscultation anteriorly nothing abnormal, but posteriorly respiratory murmurs are harsh and shrill, with occasional sibilation. At the base on right side there is crepitation on inspiration ; on the left side respiration is tubular. Vocal resonance equal superiorly and anteriorly, but posteriorly everywhere increased, on the left side amounting to bronchophony. Pulse 96, weak ; heart sounds normal ; skin hot, moderately dry, but there has been profuse perspiration ; there is dull pain in lumbar regions ; urine opaque from the existence of a reddish cloud ; sp. gr. 1024, not coagulable, but clears on the addition of heat ; chlorides diminished in quantity. ℞ Sp. Æther. Nit. ʒiij ; Potass. Acetat. ʒij ; Aquam ad ℥vj. M. One table-spoonful to be taken every four hours. ℞ Liquor. Sodæ Chlor. ℥j ; Sp. Vini Gallic. ʒss ; Infus. Rosæ. e. ad. ℥vj. M. Ft. gargarisma.

PROGRESS OF THE CASE.—*December 11th.*—Crepitation more diffused over right back. On left side respirations still dry and harsh. Chlorides absent from urine. *Dec. 12th.*—Crepitation now audible over left back. Lithates in urine more abundant. Discharge of saliva still copious, but greatly diminished in amount. Pulse 80, weak. *Habeat Vini* ℥iij *per diem. Dec. 13th.*—Chlorides in urine again perceptible. *Dec. 14th.*—Chlorides in urine abundant. Crepitation

* Reported by Mr. John Glen, Clinical Clerk.

posteriorly diminishing, sputum still copious, frothy, and somewhat gelatinous. Breath continues to give off the mercurial factor. *Dec.* *15th.*—Last night had copious diaphoresis, followed by great relief in his breathing. Still a few crepitations posteriorly, increased vocal resonance, more marked on left than on right side. Urates very abundant in urine. Convalescent. From this time he gradually improved. On the 21st all moist rale had disappeared, but respiratory murmurs harsh posteriorly, and vocal resonance still increased. *Dec.* *26th.*—Still a coppery taste in the mouth. Yesterday felt hungry for the first time, and was ordered an egg for breakfast and steak for dinner. From this time he rapidly recovered, and he was dismissed January 2, 1856.

Commentary.—In this decided case of pneumonia, with absence of chlorides from the urine, we had an opportunity of observing the effects of mercurial salivation on the progress of the disease. If it be contrasted with many other cases of the same kind previously recorded, it will be seen that the disease itself was in no way shortened by the exhibition of mercury. Resolution commenced on the 14th, but was not completed till the twenty-first day. On the other hand, the unpleasant effects produced by the mercury, the severe swelling of the tongue, soreness of the gums, and profuse salivation, must not only be regarded as so many increased evils and unnecessary symptoms superadded to the original disease, but as being the cause of prolonging the convalescence. For although the leading physical signs had disappeared on the twenty-first day, he could not eat until the twenty-sixth day, in consequence of the coppery taste in his mouth. But as soon as nutrients could be taken, he recovered rapidly. No fact could better demonstrate the utter uselessness of the drug, and its occasional mischievous effects.

CASE X.*—*Double Pneumonia—Critical Diarrhœa on the twenty-first day—Recovery.*

HISTORY.—James M'Naughton, æt. 34—admitted June 30, 1854, a shoemaker. States that he has been much addicted to the use of intoxicating liquors. From the 21st to the 23d inst. he was in a continuous state of intoxication, and on the morning of the 24th he awoke with dull pain in the chest, great dyspnœa, cough, and expectoration of matter, which, he says, resembled pure blood. He has undergone no medical treatment.

---

* Reported by Mr. Almaric Seymour, Clinical Clark.

Symptoms on Admission.—On admission, the respirations are 44 in the minute. Sputum copious, of deep prune-juice colour. On percussing the chest anteriorly, there is slight dulness on the right side inferiorly, but posteriorly the dulness is very marked over the inferior 3-4ths of both lungs. On auscultation, dry tubular breathing is heard over the dull parts, with bronchophony, but on taking a forced inspiration, coarse crepitation, deep-seated, is audible; respiration at both apices and over chest anteriorly puerile. Pulse 120, weak. Tongue covered with a yellowish fur, thirst, no appetite, headache; general appearance sallow—indicative of exhaustion; he complains of great weakness. Urine of deep cherry-red colour, sp. gr. 1020, contains no albumen or sediment, and no chlorides. Other functions normal. To have one-third of a grain of Antim. Tart. every three hours; ʒiv of wine daily.

Progress of the Case.—July 3d.—The wine was increased to ℥vj daily, his symptoms having undergone no change. July 4th.—To-day chlorides have appeared in small quantity in the urine, which presents the same cherry-red colour. Crepitation audible in left lung posteriorly, right lung as before. Sputum lighter, with less of the prune-juice appearance. July 7th.—Since last report there has been marked improvement. To-day the urine contains abundant chlorides. Crepitation over both sides of chest posteriorly. To have forty minims of Sp. Æther. Nit. and twenty grains of Potass. Acet. in solution thrice daily. July 10th.—Over the whole of back posteriorly coarse crepitation; still bronchophony, and abundant sputum tinged with blood. July 15th.— Last night was seized with diarrhœa. He had six copious watery stools. To-day no crepitation audible; respirations natural, except in left supra-scapular region, where bronchophony is still audible, but not so harsh as formerly. Urine now clear and in every way normal. Convalescent. From this day he rapidly improved, and was dismissed, August 2d, quite well.

Commentary.—This was a very severe case of double pneumonia, in a broken-down and dissipated individual, who was saved by wine, and in whom a choleraic diarrhœa, accompanied by vomiting, proved critical on the twenty-first day. The consideration of this and the previous cases must show that what really delays and prolongs convalescence is general exhaustion, and that it is of little moment how this is accomplished—whether by starvation, blood-letting, mercurials which destroy appetite, previous disease, or dissipation. Perhaps starvation is the one which is most readily overcome,

---

* Reported by Messrs. Geo. Robertson and E. P. Ritchie, Clinical Clerks.

CASE XI.*—*Acute Pericarditis followed by Acute double Pneumonia —Recovery—Aortic Incompetence—Subsequent Articular Rheumatism—Sudden Death—Adherent Pericardium—Fatty Enlarged Heart—Thickening of Aortic Valves.*

HISTORY.—Jessie Douglas, æt. 22, employed in a paper warehouse —admitted November 19th, 1855. Has never been very healthy ; has had several attacks of rheumatic fever, the last being about seven years ago. On the 9th current, after exposure to cold and damp, she was seized with rigors and pain in the back. These disappearing, were succeeded by pain and slight swelling of the knees, lasting only for a few days. During all this time, though ill, she had no headache, vomiting, nor pain in the chest, but the shortness of breath and palpitation to which she is subject became aggravated. She was under medical treatment, and got purgative medicines, but was neither bled nor leeched.

SYMPTOMS ON ADMISSION.—Apex beats distinctly between the fourth and fifth ribs, immediately under and a little to the inside of the nipple ; heart's impulse is heaving, and sensibly moves the whole momma : it can be felt but very indistinctly in the normal position ; there is no thrill. Transverse dulness at the level of the nipple 4¾ inches. Heart sounds are exceedingly indistinct, and muffled at the apex, but no murmur is heard here. At the base the first sound is almost inaudible, but with the second there is heard a soft blowing murmur. Pulse 80, full, regular, incompressible. Breathing is rather laboured ; respirations are 34 per minute, but regular ; there is slight cough and no sputum. Percussion is everywhere good ; vocal resonance is greater under the left than under the right clavicle ; no rale is audible, but respiration is exaggerated under the right clavicle and inspiration is blowing under the left. She speaks languidly, does not sleep, and on sitting up feels faint. She is thirsty, and has no appetite ; the bowels are open ; catamenia are regular. Urine is natural, sp. gr. 1016, not albuminous ; deposits copious urates and phosphates ; contains no chlorides. Patient lies on her back ; cheeks rather flushed ; the skin warm and perspiring ; no pain nor swelling of any joints. *Ordered half an ounce every fourth hour of the following :—*℞ *Liquor. Ammon. Acetat. et Aqua* ãã ʒij.

PROGRESS OF THE CASE.—*November 20th.*—At the apex, the cardiac sounds continue exceedingly indistinct and muffled. At the base, immediately above the nipple, there is heard with each cardiac sound an exceedingly soft blowing noise, equal in intensity and duration ; it extends over a considerable space, being heard but very feebly under the right nipple. Immediately under the centre of both clavicles there is a prolonged blowing noise, occupying the period of both sounds. Pulse 72, full and somewhat jerking ; palpitations are occasionally urgent ; respirations 36, laboured. *Ordered twelve leeches to be applied* over the præcordia, and subsequently warm fomentations. 21st.—The leech-bites bled well. There is great heaving and expansive motion of the whole præcordia ; at the apex, murmurs are indistinct—at the base a double blowing murmur, most clear over the head of the sternum. There is no friction audible—no pain, and the palpitations are not increased. Pulse 80, slightly jerking, but weak. She cannot sit up from tendency to faint ; is depressed and exhausted in her aspect. Urine scanty ; still contains no chlorides. *Ordered three ounces of wine with beef-tea ; to be kept perfectly quiet.* 22d.—The skin is covered with moisture ; respirations 46 ; pulse 84 ; still jerking and weak. The apex beats exactly under the fifth rib, a little to the inside of the nipple. At the base there is now a loud creaking which is double, and very loud at the margin of the sternum. Transverse dulness 3¼ inches. *Ordered to discontinue the saline mixture.* In the evening loud friction was audible at the apex as well as at the base, and the apex beat had fallen about two lines below and to the inner side. 23d.—Pulse 72, of same character ; respirations 35. At the base of the cardiac organ, instead of the double friction heard yesterday, there is now a single continuous creaking. The same sound is audible at the apex. 24th.—Pulse 80, still slightly jerking, but soft ; respirations 36 ; apex as yesterday. There is a continuous churning friction at base ; at the apex it is heard, but less loud and continuous. *R. Spir. Æther. Nitrici* ʒiij ; *Tinct. Colchici* ʒj ; *Aquæ* ʒvss ; *M. One ounce thrice a-day.* Also R. *Pulv. Opii* gr. iij ; *Extract. Catechu* gr. xv ; *Confect. Rosar. q. s. ut fiat massa in pilulas sex dividenda ; one to be taken every sixth hour.* 25th.—The same friction murmur ; pulse 80 ; respirations 36 ; urine is hyperlithic, and still contains no chlorides. 26th.—Pulse 82, slightly jerking, more compressible ; respirations 32 ; skin dry and hot ; tongue moist ; has no appetite ; urine the same in character ; the friction is less churning and continuous, and occurs more with the first sound.

November 28th.—Has had an increase of feverish symptoms for the last two or three nights, and last night she complained of cold, and required extra bed-clothes. At the visit to-day, dulness is detected in the left scapular region near the inferior angle, over a space the size of the hand, with crepitation and pealing vocal resonance. Harsh respiration over both lungs anteriorly, with sibilation and sonorous rale on expiration. There is cough, with gelatinous rusty expectoration. Friction in cardiac region is now diminishing both in intensity and duration. *Ordered three additional ounces of wine.* (From this day commenced an attack of pneumonia, affecting one-half of the left lung, terminating in seven days. Besides dulness, crepitation, and increased vocal resonance, there were on the fourth and fifth days a friction murmur at the base of the left lung.) The chlorides began to reappear in the urine on the fourth day. *A blister was applied (3 in. by 4) to the right side anteriorly on the 29th, and one of the same size to the left lateral region on Dec. 2d.* Dec. 2d.—On percussion, the transverse cardiac dulness measures 3½ inches transversely ; the apex beats feebly between the fifth and sixth ribs. At the base, one long rough prolonged sound is heard, and at the level of the nipple this is plainly connected with a second of a friction character. Over the centre of the sternum, on a level with the nipple, this hoarse blowing (or friction ?) is loudest, and is still audible at the right of the sternum within 1½ inch of the right nipple. Still dulness on percussion over inferior half of left lung posteriorly, with crepitation and ægophonic vocal resonance on auscultation. Respirations 40 in the minute. Pulse 96, still jerking and soft. *Dec. 6th.*—Considerable dulness is detected to-day on the right side from the inferior angle of scapula to the base. Respiration is almost inaudible, and is faintly bronchial. Over new area of dulness a little fine crepitation may be detected on inspiration, and vocal resonance is increased. Pulse 126, soft, jerking ; respirations 52 ; great dyspnœa. *Dec. 8th.*—Dulness now extends over two-thirds of the right lung posteriorly, where respiration is tubular, with pealing resonance of the voice. Expectoration scanty, gelatinous, and orange-coloured. Cough suppressed ; pulse 132, soft. Still rheumatic pains in left thumb and wrist. Urine loaded with urates. ℞ *Sp. Æth. Nit.*; *Potass. Acet. aā* 5ij ; *Aquam ad* ʒvj. *M. Two table-spoonfuls to be taken every four hours.* *Dec. 10th.*—The cardiac friction murmur has totally disappeared from the apex.' [At the base a blowing murmur is now heard with the second sound, the first being free from murmur. Returning crepitation heard over the lower half of right back, and above bronchial breathing. Expectoration frothy and purulent ; respirations 44 in the minute, laboured. Pulse 120, soft, but jerking. Great prostration. *Dec. 13th.*—Crepitation disappeared from right back and respiration easier. Still dulness and increased vocal resonance on left back, and respiratory murmur harsh. Tongue clean ; appetite increasing. Sweats profusely. *Was ordered ʒiv of steak.*

26th.—Since last report has been gradually gaining strength. This morning, about 9.30, the patient having assumed the recumbent position for a few minutes, violent palpitations came on, and forced her to sit up ; she felt as if about to faint, and was so agitated as to be almost unconscious. At 11 A.M., the palpitation had somewhat subsided, but the cardiac action was still very violent, shaking the whole person, and causing severe pain in the chest. Pulse almost continuous, beating about 180 times in a minute, jerking, and incompressible ; no difficulty of breathing ; no affection of the head ; face pale and anxious ; patient restless, and occasionally moaning. The urine passed soon after this paroxysm is scanty, of brick colour, turbid, clears up on application of heat, but on further heating and being fully acidified, a slight coagulum is obtained. From this paroxysm she recovered towards the evening, under the use of *Ammoniated Tincture of Valerian* and *Sol. Mur. Morphiæ.* 31st.—Patient now sits up for about two hours every day, and begins to be very hungry. *January 1st.*—Cardiac signs are the same as at last report ; at the apex nothing but a dull impulse is heard ; at the base there is still the blowing with the second sound. From this date she

H

gradually increased in strength, moving about in the ward and occasionally taking walks in the town. The pulse 90 to 100 per minute; was easily raised to 100 or 120 by excitement. Palpitations also were readily caused by any surprise, lasting for about fifteen minutes, and accompanied by a marked soreness along the sternum. On the 15th of February it is reported no change in the cardiac sounds had occurred. The transverse dulness 2¼ inches; the pulse 96, full and regular, retains its jerking character. Is discharged much relieved on the 17th February.

She was readmitted (under the care of Dr. Christison) on the 29th of February, labouring under an attack of articular rheumatism; she gradually became convalescent, but continued weak, easily agitated, with painful palpitations and threatening of syncope. The blowing murmur with the second sound at the base continued, but the most careful examination, by inspection, percussion, or auscultation, failed to elicit any other physical sign, the dulness being 3½ inches across. In this condition she continued in the ward, moving about, and in tolerable health, when on the evening of May 14th she suddenly started up with a cry, and immediately fell back, pale, gasping, and almost pulseless, and expired within three minutes, notwithstanding the sedulous administration of restoratives and stimulants.

Sectio Cadaveris—Thirty-nine hours after death.

THORAX.—The pericardium was found universally adherent. The heart was uniformly enlarged, weighing twenty-eight ounces. On pressing a stream of water down the aorta, it escaped very freely into the ventricle. On examination the aortic semilunar valves were found thickened and shortened. There were no vegetations on the valves. The auriculo-ventricular orifices, especially on the right side, were a little dilated. The left ventricle was very much dilated, and its walls were fully of the normal thickness. The right ventricle was of normal dimensions. The lungs were congested posteriorly and inferiorly, but were otherwise everywhere natural. The muscular substance of the heart was everywhere of a pale fawn colour, soft and easily breaking down under the finger.

ABDOMEN.—The abdominal organs were natural.

MICROSCOPIC EXAMINATION.—The pericardial adhesions were composed of well-formed areolar texture, in firm bands aggregated closely together. The substance of the heart presented all stages of the muscular fatty transformation: the fasciculi in most places being brittle and the transverse striæ obscure, while here and there fatty granules were numerous, displacing more or less of the sarcous substance.

Commentary.—This case was carefully observed for nearly a period of six months. On admission it was evident that a pericar-

ditis existed, with such distension of the pericardium that the two
diseased surfaces did not rub upon one another, so as to occasion
friction murmurs. The pulse was full and jerking, but the exact
character of the valvular lesion could not then be determined. There
was also dyspnœa, and with a view of diminishing this and other
symptoms, twelve leeches were applied, with the effect, however,
of rendering her weak and faint. Wine, nutrients, and quietude
were immediately ordered, and subsequently constituted the treatment. The following day the pericardial distension began to
diminish, and a returning friction murmur to appear. As the peri-
carditic signs decreased, the evidence of aortic incompetency became
more evident, and latterly a prolonged blowing with the second
sound at the base was the permanent sign of aortic valvular lesion.
She also suffered from two distinct attacks of pneumonia, one on
the left, and then subsequently on the right side, during the whole
of which time wine with nutrients were assiduously administered,
with the effect of conducting her favourably through these formidable complications. All who witnessed the case were satisfied
that this woman, during these two pneumonic attacks, in both
of which were present all the characteristic symptoms and physical signs of the disease, owed her life to good nourishment and
stimulants, and that the slightest approach towards an antiphlogistic treatment would have been fatal. It was further observable,
that at this time the pulse was full and jerking—many would have
called it hard—so that she presented what has frequently been
described as the symptoms of an exquisite case of pneumonia; in
short, that very group of symptoms in which writers have advised
us to bleed largely. I have myself no doubt, that such cases with
aortic disease and dyspnœa were, previous to the days of physical
diagnosis, regarded as typical examples of pneumonia, were bled
largely, and served to swell the great mortality which, as we have
previously shown, characterised a former practice. Under an
opposite treatment, however, she gradually recovered, and became
so well (though still labouring under the aortic incompetency with
tendency to palpitation), that she insisted on going out. Unfortunately
she was so imprudent as again to catch articular rheumatism, and
re-entered the Infirmary; the cardiac physical signs and symptoms,
however, remaining unchanged. She again recovered, but died

suddenly from a fatal syncope. On examination of the body, the correctness of all the facts observed was confirmed, and the nature of the case rendered perfectly clear. The two layers of the pericardium were everywhere adherent; the aortic valves were thickened and incompetent, explaining the persistence of the valvular murmur and jerking pulse ; the left ventricle was hypertrophied, as shown by percussion ; and the muscular substance of the heart was fatty, accounting for the sudden death. Of the pneumonia not a trace was found, and in numerous other instances which have fallen under my notice, morbid anatomy has demonstrated that of all the pulmonary diseases it is the one which leaves least signs of its existence afterwards. This fact has not been sufficiently attended to, although it supports the view I have so long maintained, that pneumonia is in no way to be dreaded, even when compared with bronchitis and pleurisy.

CASE XII.*—*General Acute Meningitis supervening on Pleuro-Pneumonia.*

HISTORY.—David Murray, æt. 43, a coal-heaver—admitted January 18, 1854. He has been an intemperate man, and a week previous to admission was seen by one of the pupils to be affected by delirium tremens. He now says, that on the 13th (which was the first day of thaw after frost and snow) he was much exposed to the weather while at work, but felt no ill effects until the morning of the 15th at four o'clock, when he awoke very sick, and vomited several times. He kept his bed, feeling feverish, and in the afternoon began to cough. On the morning of the 16th he experienced a sharp pain in the right chest, about three inches below the nipple, which was increased by coughing and inspiring deeply, and prevented his lying on that side. Has had no rigor nor headache.

SYMPTOMS ON ADMISSION.—On admission, respiration is impeded by interrupted inspirations, which give pain. Over the lower half of the right lung posteriorly, there is marked dulness on percussion, loud crepitation on inspiration, and bronchophony. The sputa are scanty, consisting of gelatinous matter, with rusty brown patches. No dyspnœa. Pulse 120, strong and full ; skin hot and dry ; tongue dry, furred, and fissured ; great thirst ; no appetite ; bowels open. Has no headache at present, but says he is restless at night, and sleeps badly. Other functions normal. *To have one-third of a grain of tartrate of antimony in solution every two hours.*

PROGRESS OF THE CASE.—*January 22d.*—Since last report the

pneumonia has followed its usual course. On the 20th crepitation had disappeared, but has returned to-day. Yesterday evening was ordered a diuretic draught, containing Sp. Æther. Nit. 5j. The pulse 130, weak, and at the visit his replies to questions were a little confused. *January 23d.*—Yesterday afternoon he was observed to mutter incoherently, but remained quiet until eight P.M., when he became violently delirious. He had a very wild and fierce expression of eye and countenance, insisted on getting up, would not be controlled, and struggled violently with those who endeavoured to restrain him. He spoke little, but made incoherent noises. The pupils were much dilated ; the pulse very rapid and weak. *The head was shaved, and constant cold applied.* Prostration, however, coming on, *wine and stimulants were given freely.* He continued now and then to struggle violently ; strabismus was apparent latterly. Died exhausted at 6 A.M. this morning.

Sectio Cadaveris.—Thirty-one hours after death.

Body greatly emaciated.

HEAD.—On removing the skull-cap, the dura mater presented a uniform yellowish tint, dependent on a recent exudation below it. On removal, the subarachnoid tissue was infiltrated with a soft exudation, which covered the entire surface of both hemispheres, and of the cerebellum. It was as abundant at the base as on the superior surface of the brain. On cutting into the cerebral substance, it was observed that the yellow exudation accompanied the inflexions of the pia mater between the convolutions. The lateral ventricles contained 3iss of turbid serum. The lining walls of the ventricles were a little congested ; the choroid plexuses healthy. The septum lucidum rather soft, but the other portions of the brain normal.

THORAX.—Three lower fourths of the right lung presented the characters of grey hepatisation posteriorly. The anterior surfaces were healthy. The pleura covering this lung were partially adherent, with some shreds of recent lymph. Other thoracic organs healthy.

ABDOMEN.—The liver enlarged, weighing 6 lbs. 4 oz., of pale colour, and soft. The spleen also soft and pulpy. Other abdominal organs healthy.

MICROSCOPIC EXAMINATION.—The exudation poured out in the subarachnoid cavity had everywhere undergone the transformation into pus. The turbid fluid in the lateral ventricles also contained some pus, with a few epithelial cells. The cerebral tissue was healthy. The liver cells contained an unusual amount of fatty granules. The pneumonic portion of the right lung was infiltrated with fluid molecular matter and pus corpuscles, most of which were more or less collapsed, and all of them very granular. The whole evidently in a state of disintegration.

Commentary.—In this man, who was intemperate, and labouring under pneumonia, which was progressing favourably, there

supervened at noon on the seventh day of the disease a little confusion in his ideas, which in the course of the afternoon passed
into violent delirium, causing strabismus and dilated pupils. At
night he became comatose, and died at five o'clock next morning.
At the commencement of the pneumonia he had vomited, a symp-
tom perhaps referable in him to cerebral irritation—a condition
which the febrile state he was subsequently thrown into, however,
did not appear to augment in any unusual degree. On examining
the head after death, the subarachnoid cavity and involutions of
the pia mater over the whole surface of the brain were loaded with
purulent matter, and 3iss of turbid serum was effused into the
lateral ventricles. This, therefore, was an instance of very rapid
death from meningitis, a result partly attributable to his previous
intemperate habits, and partly to the circumstance that the disease
appeared at a time when he was much exhausted by the pneumonic attack. In this, as in Case III., it is observable that the
occurrence of extensive exudation is in no way incompatible with
depression of the bodily powers, a fact altogether opposed to the
supposed connection between inflammation and a sthenic state of
the constitution. In fact, the extent as well as the fatality of the
cerebral disease is probably to be attributed to the exhaustion of
the vital powers at the time of its occurrence.
   The pneumonia went through its usual progress, and on the
day when the meningitis commenced the returning crepitation was
audible. On examination after death, the whole pulmonary exudation was found softened and converted into pus, which was already
undergoing rapid disintegration. Here, then, is the positive proof
that the returning crepitation is caused by the transformation of
the exudation into pus, and that the resolution of the disease is
owing to the disintegration and liquefaction of the pus-cells,
changes which were progressing in this case. Exactly the same
appearances may be observed whenever pneumonia is fatal at this
period, a circumstance which has satisfied me, as stated p. 49,
that grey hepatisation, instead of being the exceptional and dangerous consequence of pneumonia, is the usual process by which
the exudation is broken up and absorbed.